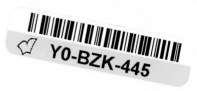

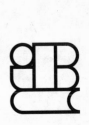

Working with Latino Youth

Culture, Development, and Context

Joan D. Koss-Chioino

Luis A. Vargas

Forewords by José Szapocznik and Lillian Comas-Díaz

Jossey-Bass Publishers • San Francisco

Jossey-Bass books and products are available through most bookstores. To contact Jossey-Bass directly, call (888) 378–2537, fax to (800) 605–2665, or visit our website at www.josseybass.com.

Substantial discounts on bulk quantities of Jossey-Bass books are available to corporations, professional associations, and other organizations. For details and discount information, contact the special sales department at Jossey-Bass.

 Manufactured in the United States of America on Lyons Falls Turin Book. This paper is acid-free and 100 percent totally chlorine-free.

Library of Congress Cataloging-in-Publication Data

Koss-Chioino, Joan.
    Working with Latino youth : culture, development, and context /
Joan D. Koss-Chioino, Luis A. Vargas ; forewords by José Szapocznik
and Lillian Comas-Díaz.
      p.   cm.
    Includes bibliographical references and index.
    ISBN 0-7879-4325-8
    1. Hispanic American youth—Mental health.   2. Hispanic American
youth—Mental health services. I. Vargas, Luis A.
II. Title.
RC451.5.H57K67   1999
616.89'0089'68073—dc21   99-22758

FIRST EDITION
HB Printing 10 9 8 7 6 5 4 3 2

Contents

Foreword I

While some cultural groups are concerned with the self, Latino people are deeply engaged with their social and cultural contexts. It is therefore not surprising that a contextualist perspective—which views context as the weaving together of the individual and his or her social fabric—would explain a contextualist people so well. In contrast to European psychology's early love affair with self-oriented intrapersonal processes and American psychology's modernistic attachment to individually oriented self-actualization and autonomy, postmodern perspectives on adolescent development are interested in the influence of social and cultural contexts on children's developmental trajectories.

A contextualist perspective, like behavioral genetics, is characterized by an interest in understanding the diversity of patterns of the human condition as well as recognizing the heterogeneity within those patterns. Such a perspective has an exquisite ability to recognize how apparently small variations in context can produce markedly different results. Take the case of children in the same family. Although siblings share considerable genetic, social, and cultural antecedents, there is enough variability between siblings for each to be remarkably different from the other.

Similarly, the authors of this book remark on the considerable differences among people of Latino ancestry. Latinos are a complex mosaic of people who have been exposed to a broad range of cultural streams and social contexts and today constitute a heterogeneous constellation of groups. Recognizing that fact, this book is a plea against the stereotyping of Latinos and a call for recognition of the considerable uniqueness of each Latino youth and family and each Latino group.

The marriage between anthropology and clinical psychology succeeds in this book better than ever before. The collaboration of an anthropologist and a psychologist has brought a fresh look to the contextualist inclination of a people and keen insight into the kind of professional thinking that permits us to work with contextually focused clients. The book reaffirms the fundamental role of families in the Latino context. It explores the role of social and cultural context in influencing families as a group or differentially through its members. It depicts the role of therapists as interwoven into the sociocultural fabric of the client. And it discusses the broader sociocultural and political issues that influence people in relation to their impact on our clinical work with Latino youth.

Working with Latino Youth is an inspiring book. It inspires the clinician to be humble in the process of discovery about a client. It teaches the clinician to explore the social, cultural, and contextual worlds of the client—rather than the client's having to adjust to the unfamiliar experience of therapy, the therapist must learn to fit into the client's world. The therapist does this by behaving in ways that reflect an understanding that individuals are integral parts of the many environments in which they interact and that historical environmental processes have shaped their current experiences and behaviors.

At another level this book tells the story of a people whose ancestry reflected the adage that the whole village raises the child. Latino culture originated in agrarian indigenous societies in which small and complex kinship networks were effective in the management of small-scale food production. Shaped by the values of traditional agricultural communities, Latinos today find themselves in a very complex set of connected but uncoordinated social processes. They have been deeply affected by the altered patterns of relationships among adults and between children and their adult relatives and neighbors that have resulted from the vast changes that have occurred over time. The authors teach us how to understand and help such people. The message is simple: listen to the client, and be attentive to the client's circumstances, past and present.

Miami, Florida   JOSÉ SZAPOCZNIK
March 1999

Foreword II

The Latino experience is a metaphor for our country's development. Latino youngsters transform their identities while remaining true to their roots. Don Quixote's words, "I want to be someone else without ceasing to be myself," seem to characterize Latino identity development. *Working with Latino Youth: Culture, Development, and Context* offers a comprehensive approach for clinical intervention. Using two paradigms—ecological development and social constructionism—Joan D. Koss-Chioino and Luis A. Vargas successfully develop a practice model that adequately centers culture and development within psychological interventions. Anchoring their approach in theory that highlights the individual-in-context, these authors follow Ortega y Gasset's dictum *"Yo soy yo y mis circumstancias"* (I am me and my circumstances) and thus remain culturally valid and ethical.[1] Acknowledging the interrelationhips of linked contexts such as family, peers, school, community, and street life, they stress the relevance of environmental fit in working with Latino youngsters.

Serving as extraordinary guides illuminating a path in our national peregrination, Koss-Chioino and Vargas recognize that ethnicity is a process and that culture is development. Following these principles, they prophesy the hybridization of North America through the emergence of its "new ethnic minority." Accordingly, as unmeltable ethnics, Latinos bear a hyphenated identity, transforming their environment into cultural borderlands. This process threatens the national (white) identity and generates anti-immigrant positions, English-only movements, and anti–affirmative action positions. Nonetheless, the Latino presence is stronger than ever; for instance, Mexican immigration accounts for the largest number of immigrants from one country to the United States in recent history.[2] Such a demographic avalanche is contributing to what Eva Hoffman calls our number one concern—a national identity problem.[3] Indeed, the advisory board to the U.S. President's Commission on Race has declared that the greatest challenge facing Americans today is to accept and take pride in defining ourselves as a multiracial democracy.

Latinos' experience serves as a compass in our national redefinition because their odyssey parallels the progress of the United States. Historically, some Latinos were natives to this land; others arrived searching for the immigrant dream or the Golden Fleece of opportunities and freedom; and still others continue to be washed up on American shores searching for political and religious asylum. Their journey—paved with discrimination, socioeconomic challenge, trauma, and cultural adjustment—is emblematic of our national aspiration, *E pluribus unum* (Out of many, one).

Working with Latino Youth canvasses an ethnic mosaic, casting the "melting pot" as an *arpillera,* the brilliant tapestry woven by Latin Americans as a response to oppression. Like an *arpillera,* this therapeutic model considers the historical and political contexts as integral components of functioning, identifying oppression as a psychological reality. Like an *arpillera,* it creates beauty out of pain and meaning out of chaos. Moreover, Latinos' ability to recover from pain, trauma, and oppression is impressive and inspiring. As an illustration, "Nuyorican" poets define the transformation of aggression into strength among oppressed people as a "dusmic" process.[4] The dusmic spirit prevails among many Latinos, growing out of desperation and a genuine self-affirmation. As Dadi Piñero articulates, the dusmic spirit gives hope without deceptive illusions:

> Now is now
> What happened happened
> and what's starting now
> is beginning and what's past
> has ended and what's ahead of us
> will be the end.[5]

Although Latino youngsters are a "population at risk," they are resilient, resourceful, and creative. The fact that Mexican immigrants have better mental health profiles than people of Mexican descent born in the United States seems consistent with the belief that traditional culture has protective effects because it may contribute to healthier habits leading to better health.[6] Latinos' multiculturalism, pluralism, and adaptability can become building blocks in assembling the "One America" that the President's Commission on Race aspires to. *Working with Latino Youth* documents Latino resistance and creative responses to oppression. Its emphasis on protective and dusmic factors challenges deficit models of culture and ethnicity. Koss-Chioino and Vargas's decision to introduce each chapter with a rap couplet by a Latino former gang member who is now a productive member of society is emblematic of their approach. They rescue the value of traditional cultures by discussing indigenous resources, overcoming adversity, and celebrating syncretism. Combining psychology, ethnographic methods, and anthropology, they offer psychological tools such as profiling and taking individuals' environmental context into consideration. Likewise, they redefine the clinician's role as inquirer, collaborator, and negotiator, present vivid case material, and provide excellent clinical guidelines for intervention.

Koss-Chioino and Vargas's model can be aptly applied to other youth of color and to all youngsters regardless of ethnicity. By rescuing cultural practices, strengthening dusmic spirits, and delivering culturally consonant services, this contextual model remains grounded in ecological and psychological templates that expand the lens of our traditional psychological theory and practice. *Working with Latino Youth* takes the field a step further, to a place where ecology, psychology, culture, development, and anthropology converge—creating and re-creating a healing *arpillera*.

Washington, D.C.   LILLIAN COMAS-DÍAZ
March 1999

Notes

1. Ortega y Gasset, J. *Man and Crisis* (New York: Norton, 1958).
2. Escobar, J. "Commentary: Immigration and Mental Health: Why Are Immigrants Better Off?" *Archives of General Psychiatry, 55*(9) (1998): 781–782.
3. Hoffman, E. *Lost in Translation: A Life in a New Language* (New York: Penguin, 1989).
4. Algarón, M., and Piñero, M. (eds.). *Nuyorican Poetry: An Anthology of Puerto Rican Words and Feelings* (New York: Morrow, 1975).
5. Algarón and Piñero, *Nuyorican Poetry*, p. 85.
6. Escobar, "Commentary."

To our families

Craig, Rhea, Judith, Hugh, and goddaughter Zaira
—JDK-C

   and

Janet, Kate, and Elizabeth
—LAV

Preface

Despite a growing literature on how to conduct psychological interventions with ethnically diverse children and adolescents, few works integrate development, culture, and psychological intervention. Although efforts to make clinical practice "culturally competent" (to use the latest term in vogue) continue, many practitioners remain dissatisfied with the adequacy of the suggested modifications to current practice models. We believe that one of the reasons for this dissatisfaction is that the suggested modifications are still largely based on current theories that do not allow for the incorporation of culture and development in clinical formulations and subsequent intervention strategies. The solution to making psychological interventions culturally and developmentally responsive is not to continue to modify existing practice models based on theories that decontextualize the individual—that ignore the "local worlds" in which the individual participates. We believe that the solution to developing practice models that adequately consider culture and development as integral to psychological intervention is to base intervention on theory that highlights the individual-in-context. In this book, we present a contextual approach to psychological interventions with a focus on Latino youth.

This book represents a mutual and equal collaboration between a medical anthropologist and a clinical psychologist applied to the task of making psychological interventions culturally and developmentally responsive to Latino youth. Our collaboration, begun in an earlier edited volume in 1992, brought together two different perspectives on youths as cultural and psychological beings. Anthropology allowed us to view the experience of Latino youth from the perspective of their local worlds, provided a methodological approach to acquiring knowledge about those worlds, and gave us an attitude of humility with regard to what practitioners need to know about their clients. We delved into the many threads of the tapestry of psychology in order to arrive at a template for clinical practice in which cultural and developmental processes are salient. Toward this end, we explored recent theories in developmental and clinical child psychology, social constructivism, and ecological psychology. Our model for psychological intervention falls within what would be considered in epistemology as contextualism and synthesizes developmental and cultural theories.

In writing this book, we had to confront the issue of what we mean by *Latino*. The term does a disservice to our young clients and their families in that it takes away an important cultural identity and replaces it with an all-encompassing label that masks the contexts that clinical practitioners need to experience with their clients. This dilemma represents the initial struggle we faced in writing a book about culture, development, and psychological intervention. We debated whether we should limit the coverage to one loosely defined cultural group. Would such limited coverage decrease the applicability of the book to other ethnic groups? In the end, we decided to address a population that is currently described as Latino but that in actuality encompasses diverse cultures and ethnic groups. We did so in part because these are the groups with which we work most frequently and in part because of our own life experiences, spending formative years in Puerto Rico (JDKC) and growing up as a Mexican American in the Southwest (LAV).

Having decided to limit the book to the area of our most significant experiences, we questioned if an approach to intervention with Latinos is applicable to other cultural groups. For this answer we only needed to look around us. In a recent presentation at a national conference by past psychology interns in which one of us participated, there were a Czechoslovakian-Haitian raised in Montreal, an American Indian–Venezuelan raised in a Greek Orthodox family, and a Jewish American man married to an Indian woman of the Zoroastrian faith. And we looked at Latino staff at a research center in the Southwest, which included a Mexican woman raised in the United States married to a recent Colombian immigrant, a Puerto Rican woman raised in Puerto Rico whose ex-husband is Nicaraguan, a woman from a European Jewish family who was raised in Argentina, and an American-Spanish woman. It is not just the one-tenth of the U.S. population represented as "Hispanics" or the one-fourth represented as "ethnic minorities" that we as practitioners must be concerned about. The United States is rapidly becoming a hybridized nation composed of people with mixed cultural backgrounds—what we might call the new ethnic majority! How can practitioners deal with this new level of diversity? Although the approach we describe addresses Latinos specifically, it is intended to present practitioners with a model that can be applied to diverse cultural groups because of its contextual orientation.

Audience

Working with Latino Youth is intended for mental health practitioners, including clinical, counseling, and school psychologists, psychiatrists, and social workers; counselors, public health administrators, and planners; and mental health agency administrators who work with or administrate programs for culturally diverse children, adolescents, and families. This book describes in depth an approach to intervening with youths in the contexts of their environments. Although we do not offer techniques for working with specific problems, we do offer considerable detail on how to assess problems and target solutions within an approach that views culture as integral to clinical work.

Organization of the Book

Chapter One describes the need to take a contextual view in working with Latino youth. This chapter first presents a demography of Latino populations and then explores the distinction between culture and ethnicity, as well as ethnicity as a process. It concludes with an examination of the implications of Latino social traditions and historical contexts.

Chapter Two presents a contextual theory on how to develop psychosocial approaches to treatment that are responsive to both culture and development. Although we consider our perspective essential to the development of effective psychological interventions in general, it is especially important for ethnic children and adolescents, who may be the least understood. This chapter sets the stage for our discussion of child and adolescent development across Latino cultural groups and its relationship to emotional and behavioral problems that youth experience.

Chapter Three examines the activities of an individual within one context, such as family, school, and peer group. In this chapter, we explore relationships within immediate environments—or microsystems—in which Latino youth live. We discuss parenting practices and spirituality in the family environment of Latino youth. We also discuss the role of language, the sense of self, and ethnic and racial socialization at this level of analysis.

Chapter Four is clinical in scope and presents clinical case studies of youth with behavioral and emotional problems associated with one or more of the contexts described in Chapter Three. We examine the conceptualization of the presenting problem and how solutions to the problem must consider the individual's functioning in daily activity settings. We describe how assessment and treatment can be conducted from a contextualist perspective in which the therapist collaborates with clients and their families.

Interrelationships among linked contexts, such as between family and peers, family and school, school and street life, are the focus of Chapter Five. This chapter discusses the concepts of risk and environmental fit. Assessment and intervention in linked contexts, such as family and school and peer groups and family, are described. This chapter highlights how life choices are assessed and valued by parents and other socializing agents. In addition, issues around personal and ethnic identity, acculturation, and immigration are discussed.

Like Chapter Four, Chapter Six is clinical in scope. It presents case material related to the problems and issues raised in Chapter Five. It also details techniques for assessment and intervention, based in part on ethnographic method, and specifies the clinician's role as that of inquirer, collaborator, and negotiator.

Chapter Seven focuses on major institutions and settings such as the community in relation to family, school, and peer-group activities. It discusses changes in mental health practices toward community-based interventions and how community standards and regulations affect these practices. It also examines issues that affect mental health practice at a community level, such as the ways in which youth and adult subcultures are created, the ways in which experiences are transmitted across generations, and ethnic identity conflict and poverty.

Chapter Eight focuses on how cultural orientations contextualize individual lifescapes and includes broader arenas, such as U.S. society and Latino countries of origin. It explores the role of various cultural orientations in interventions with Latino youth as the broadest context of activities relevant to a number of themes that are essential to an understanding of how problem behavior develops and how this understanding is central to the formulation of developmentally and culturally appropriate interventions.

In the final chapter, Chapter Nine, we discuss the implications of our model for developing interventions from a contextual perspective. We explore how managed care structures the way interventions are formulated and delivered and the danger of the failure to take cultural diversity into account. We examine how the paradigms from which interventions are derived determine the extent to which cultural diversity is addressed. Finally, we describe how contextual perspectives change the focus of evaluating treatment outcomes.

Acknowledgments

We have been fortunate to have a very stimulating, bright, and talented group of students, psychology interns, and clinical research staff, as well as some very special colleagues (among whom are Louise Baca, Artemio Brambila, Lydia Buki, José M. Cañive, John Gutierrez, Mary Kaven, Vesna Kutlesic, Ricardo Martinez, Cynthia Nemeth, Beatriz Ramirez, Fredeswinda Roman, Bradley Samuel, Julienne Smrcka, and Diana M. Valdez), who have helped us clarify our ideas. We also wish to thank Elizabeth Rahdert, program officer at the National Institute on Drug Abuse (Treatment Branch), who administered and commented on the Arizona treatment research that formed a significant part of the background to this work. We owe a special debt of gratitude to our spouses, Craig C. Chioino and Janet Hodde-Vargas, and children, Kate and Elizabeth Vargas, for their patience, tolerance, and support during late nights and missed weekends. We also are deeply appreciative of our young clients and their families who, in the midst of turmoil, were tolerant of our blunders and helped us understand them.

We especially thank Placido Vasquez Jr. for allowing us to use rap verses that he composed as a teenager back in 1989, when he was a member of a gang. Now a successful college student working on a prelaw degree, he graciously allowed us to benefit from the creativity that arose out of a difficult period in his life journey.

We much appreciate the work of Sylvia Jones, who helped prepare the final version of the manuscript. Finally, we thank Alan Rinzler and Katie Levine at Jossey-Bass, as well as an anonymous reader, whose feedback helped us produce a better book.

March 1999   JOAN D. KOSS-CHIOINO
                                                       Tempe, Arizona

                                                       LUIS A. VARGAS
                                                       Albuquerque, New Mexico

The Authors

JOAN D. KOSS-CHIOINO is professor of anthropology and an affiliate of the Women's Studies Program at Arizona State University, Tempe, where she developed and currently directs the Program in Medical Anthropology. She is also visiting professor in the Department of Psychiatry and Neurology, Tulane Medical Center, and has taught at Mahidol University, Selaya, Thailand.

Koss-Chioino received her Ph.D. degree (1965) in anthropology from the University of Pennsylvania and held a postdoctoral fellowship in psychiatry and medical anthropology at the University of California Medical Center, San Francisco (1974–1976).

Koss-Chioino teaches and researches at the interface between anthropology, psychiatry, and psychology. Her primary research interest is the treatment—whether traditional, alternative, or psychotherapeutic—of illness and emotional problems in Latino cultures in the United States, Latin America, Spain, and Thailand. Currently, she is concluding a treatment research project with problem behavior and drug-abusing Mexican and Mexican American youths and families in Arizona, funded by the National Institute on Drug Abuse, and plans to carry out a community study of how older women in Spain resist depression.

Her publications include *Women as Healers, Women as Patients: Mental Health Care and Traditional Healing in Puerto Rico* (Westview Press, 1992) and *Working with Culture: Psychotherapeutic Interventions with Ethnic Minority Children and Adolescents* (Jossey-Bass, 1992), edited with Luis A. Vargas.

LUIS A. VARGAS is director of the Clinical Child Psychology Internship Program and associate professor in the Division of Child and Adolescent Psychiatry, Department of Psychiatry, University of New Mexico Health Sciences Center. He is also director of psychology at the University of New Mexico Children's Psychiatric Hospital.

Vargas received his B. A. degree (1973) in psychology from St. Edward's University in Austin, Texas; his M.S. degree (1976) in psychology from Trinity University in San Antonio, Texas; and his Ph.D. degree (1982) in clinical psychology from the University of Nebraska–Lincoln. He completed a predoctoral internship (1979) at the Neuropsychiatric Institute, University of California at Los Angeles, Center for Health Sciences, and a postdoctoral fellowship (1983) at the University of Southern California Institute of Psychiatry, Law, and Behavioral Science.

Vargas's main clinical and research interests are cultural issues in the assessment and treatment of children, adolescents, and families; training psychologists and other mental health professionals to provide culturally and developmentally responsive mental health services to children, adolescents, and their families; treatment of seriously emotionally disturbed children; schizophrenic-spectrum disorders in children; treatment of Latino youth at risk for delinquency and substance abuse; and bereavement following violent death.

Chapter One

Arenas for Therapeutic Intervention

All across America, creating this hysteria,
It's all about an area and which one's superior.
PLACIDO VASQUEZ JR.

In our previous book, *Working with Culture,* we suggested that the experience of culturally diverse children and adolescents in psychotherapy with a therapist of the dominant culture is akin to Alice's encounter with the Red Queen in Lewis Carroll's *Through the Looking Glass.*[1] The first time she meets the Red Queen, Alice tells her that she has lost her way. Rather annoyed, the Red Queen impatiently replies that all the ways around there belong to her. Like Alice, these young clients are confronted by therapists who, behaving like the Red Queen, fail to understand and appreciate their clients' experiences and perspectives. The problem, which we have called *the Red Queen phenomenon,* arises not only because psychotherapy is culturally based but also because many therapeutic interventions for children and adolescents have been adapted from adult models.

The Red Queen phenomenon represents a failure to consider both culture and development in treating youth. The general goal of this book is to help mental health professionals become culturally responsive in their work with youth from diverse Latino subcultures in the United States. The specific aim is to develop a *contextual approach* to working with Latino children, adolescents, and their families that emphasizes the integration of development and culture into psychological interventions.

1

The contextual model that we describe draws from two recent theoretical paradigms that have given rise to innovative practice models. *Developmental ecology,* the first paradigm, focuses on the social contexts within which a person interacts. These social contexts range from the immediate environment, such as the family, to remote environments, such as North American society.[2] From this perspective, problems and their solutions are viewed as situated in the interactions between an individual and social contexts. Thus, the arena for psychological intervention is greatly expanded. *Social constructionism,* the second paradigm, stresses that because development is socially constructed within local communities a person cannot be understood outside of the context of his or her history and culture.[3] This perspective draws attention to how clients' lives are influenced by social and political processes that also contextualize the therapeutic process. Although we focus on various subcultures within the Latino population in the United States, the theories and practice guidelines presented in this book are applicable to working with a wide spectrum of ethnic minority youth.

The approach we use in this book is based on the idea that individuals are integral parts of the many environments in which they interact. Many years ago, A. Irving Hallowell proposed a theory of the *culturally constituted behavioral environment.*[4] According to this theory, cultural traditions define the nature and characteristics of environments within which individuals live. Therefore, individuals can only respond or interact by way of the meanings that their cultures define, and these meanings change over time pursuant to important social and biological events. For example, parents in rural Mexican villages expect that neighbors, shopkeepers, and officials will share their child-rearing responsibilities. In contrast, immigrant parents quickly discover that urban community members in the United States do not expect to share child-rearing responsibilities and may even view the manifestation of such expectations as parental neglect. Yet, ironically, it is this type of traditional rural practice that troubled U.S. communities are trying to revive, as expressed in the now-popular saying, "It takes a village to raise a child."

Focusing on an individual child, as is often the practice in mental health treatment, does not address the settings in which the child is developing or reflect the experience of the developmental process from the child's, parents', teachers', or peers' viewpoints. Although all children develop a sense of their own uniqueness and desire recognition by others, their individuality is the result of interactions between their unique biological inheritance and their familial and environmental niches. Furthermore, the person each child will become is affected by the historical period in which he or she was born and the place of birth. The course of a child's development will be influenced by particular events that take place during his or her life. Definitions, expectations, values, attitudes, meanings, and even emotions associated with activities and relationships to other persons, other beings (ranging from pets to ancestral spirits or deities), and the environment are all contextualized by culture, including its expressive, social, and historical dimensions.

The life of César Chávez, a man who passionately defended the rights of migrant farmworkers, illustrates our notion of contextualization. Chávez founded the National Farm Workers Association (NFWA) in 1962, which later became the well-known and influential United Farm Workers (UFW) union. Although Chávez was unquestionably a very special person, his life circumstances and experiences also can be appreciated as clearly influenced by the timing and place of his birth, his Mexican American ethnicity, his family's culture, and his social status as the child of Mexican migrant farmworkers.

Chávez was born into a poor family in Yuma, Arizona, in 1927, just before the Great Depression.[5] As a result of being cheated out of his land, his father moved the family to California, where he worked as a migrant farmworker. Because Spanish was forbidden in the California schools at that time and the family spoke Spanish in the home, young César experienced significant language conflicts at school, as well as considerable discrimination. He rejected formal education. After the eighth grade, when his father suffered an accident, César went to work in the fields to help his family. Later in his life, education would become very central to him. He had hundreds of books on subjects ranging from philosophy, economics, and unions, to biographies of St. Francis, Gandhi, and the Kennedys. Despite his personal experience with oppression and exploitation, he passionately valued service to others and nonviolence in the struggle for civil rights of farmworkers.

César Chávez's emergence as an extraordinary leader is best understood in the context of his life experiences at a particular point in American history. Although his unique inheritance—both cultural and genetic—was important to his accomplishments, would this great man have so significantly influenced our society at another moment in time?

In this introductory chapter, we first provide demographic information about Latino populations. We then distinguish culture from ethnicity and explore ethnicity as a process, including the prevailing view toward cultural diversity in the United States. Finally, we present a historical perspective on the cultural characteristics of Latino ethnic groups.

Demographics of Latino Populations

Those persons to whom we refer by the term *Latino* come from a large variety of groups with distinct cultural traditions. It has been the current fashion and national policy, as reflected in the U.S. census, to label all these groups as *Hispanics*. Recent objectors to this term view the Hispanic label as referring only to the Spanish European legacy within Latino communities.[6] In fact, these communities also have Native American (indigenous peoples of all the Americas) or African American components, in equal or greater measure, according to group and country of origin. The perennial problem of "what's in a name" manifests poignantly with regard to ethnic identification across groups. After giving reasons why the term *Hispanic* is not a good one to identify the diverse populations that have been officially categorized as such, Dicochea and Mata note: "Above all, we must realize that being Latina or Latino is a state of mind. It is not based on the color of our skin, nor on the blood which courses through our veins. It is based on the fact that as a population we are severely underrepresented in the institutions which shape and control our lives. Being Latina/o is a consciousness which determines how we act and interact in this world."[7]

As the title of our book makes evident, we agree with the reasoning of these young authors and others, and we prefer the term *Latino,* which denotes Latin American (by contrast with North American) origin and thus lays claim to the history and legacy of that subhemisphere. However, it should be noted that we use the term *Hispanic* throughout this book when that term was used in the original source we are discussing.

There are an estimated 30,587,000 Hispanics in the United States.[8] (It should be noted that this figure may be an underestimate because of problems in accounting for undocumented persons.) About 11 percent of the total population of the United States is of Hispanic origin.[9] In 1993, Mexicans were the largest group by far, representing 64.3 percent of the total Latino population; Puerto Ricans were second with about 10.6 percent; Cubans accounted for 4.7 percent; Central and South Americans, as a group, represented 13.4 percent; and 7.0 percent were Hispanics who originated elsewhere.[10] As of 1997, 13.1 million, or one out of two, foreign-born residents in the United States was a native of Central America, South America, or the Caribbean.[11] Of these foreign-born residents, about 7 million, or some 53 percent, were from Mexico.[12] In 1997, 55.8 percent of Hispanics were born in the United States.[13]

From the perspective of a study of children and adolescents, it is significant that the Latino population is young. In 1997, fully 35.7 percent of all Hispanics were under eighteen years of age.[14] Among Latinos age twenty-five and over, five in ten had completed high school by 1994 and about 9 percent had bachelor's degrees.[15] Moreover, Hispanic groups by country of origin differed significantly in educational attainment: South Americans and Cubans were 60 to 100 percent more likely than other Hispanics to obtain bachelor's degrees. Only one-third as many Mexicans as South Americans earned college degrees.[16]

In thinking about psychological interventions, it is extremely important to know about conventions of language use, because intimate feelings are more readily expressed in an individual's first language. In 1990, 78 percent of Latinos spoke Spanish at home; about half reported that they were also fluent in English. As more recent immigrants, two-thirds of Dominicans and Central Americans reported that they did not speak English well.[17]

Family composition is another important consideration. In 1994, 68 percent of Latino families were two-parent families and 25 percent were headed by women alone.[18] Puerto Ricans and Dominicans had significantly more women-headed families (56 percent and 50 percent, respectively) than the other cultural groups, among which less than 20 percent of families were headed by women alone.[19] In 1993, 27 percent of Latino families were at or below poverty level compared with 11 percent of non-Latino families; however, the rates ranged from 17 percent for Cuban families to 35 percent for Puerto Rican families.[20] Furthermore, 41 percent of children and adolescents were poor, compared with 20 percent of non-Latino youth.[21]

Finally, geographic area and density-of-residence patterns are important because they relate both to lifestyles of families (economic opportunities, schools, social services, ethnic composition of community) and types of problems encountered in children and adolescents. Geographic area is particularly important with regard to intergroup relations between Latinos and the dominant society. According to the Census Bureau, the states with the largest Hispanic population in 1997 were as follows: California, with an estimated Hispanic population of 9.9 million, Texas with 5.7 million, New York with 2.6 million, Florida with 2.1 million, and Illinois with 1.2 million.[22] The states with the largest percentage of Hispanics were these: New Mexico (40 percent of total population), California (31 percent), Texas (29 percent), Arizona (22 percent), and Nevada (15 percent).[23]

Distinguishing Culture from Ethnicity

Although the terms *culture* and *ethnicity* are often used interchangeably, they represent different ideas. Culture refers to the ideological dimension of the human condition that guides and motivates behavior. That which is cultural is expressed in both material phenomena (such as the statue of *La Virgen de Guadalupe*) and social phenomena (such as the pilgrimages to the sites where *La Virgen* has appeared). Culture is transmitted—often in modified form—across generations. Its content consists of specific meanings (for example, values, attitudes, worldviews, and self-views) through which behavior and events are constructed, deconstructed, and reconstructed. Consider the celebration of *El Día de los Muertos* (Day of the Dead), which takes place on November 1 and 2 in many regions of Mexico. On this occasion, family members who have died are commemorated on home altars, and offerings of food and flowers are placed on their graves. This custom is a synthesis of Native American and Spanish Catholic practices that celebrates the coexistence of life and death. Among Mexican Americans in the United States, *El Día de los Muertos* has been deconstructed to a position of less importance in the community. In the last couple of decades, it has been reconstructed as a community celebration sponsored by museums and Mexican American voluntary associations.

In contrast to culture, ethnicity is a sociological distinction that refers to particular social groups in complex societies, groups differentiated not only on the basis of a range of shared cultural content but also on the bases of social attitudes and economic and political considerations. Ethnic groupings result from specific processes. The dominant society establishes boundary-setting and boundary-maintaining rules that define groups. Fredrik Barth, an anthropologist, viewed ethnicity as a process of constructing boundaries that define ethnic groups, rather than cultural content within these boundaries determining their definition.[24] For example, the term *Chicano* has come to be used as an ethnic label to differentiate people of Mexican descent born in the United States from Mexicans born in Mexico. Despite differentiation into two ethnic groups, Chicanos and Mexicans share many aspects of the ancestral culture, with the exception of incorporation of more aspects of U.S. culture on the part of Chicanos. What many Chicanos consider important is their asserting an ethnic identity that is distinct from Mexicans rather than having different beliefs and behavior.

In our view, the process by which ethnic groups define themselves complements the dominant society's efforts to establish the boundaries that identify them. Dynamic interaction between the dominant society's imposition of social difference and the group's ethnic identification creates a social context for intragroup and intergroup relationships. Since the 1970s, the efforts of Chicanos to differentiate themselves as an ethnic group based on birth and residency in the United States has paralleled the dominant society's identification of them as different from other Latinos.

Ethnicity as a Process

Many social scientists have based ethnicity on the notion of cultural difference that persists over time. They assume that immigrants carry with them the cultural guidelines of their countries of origin but subsequently undergo a unidirectional process by which they inevitably adopt aspects of the dominant culture, some more readily than others. European immigrants in 1942, prior to World War II, were expected to assimilate to American culture as the invariable result of a process of adaptation. However, since the 1970s cultural diversity has become a prevalent theme of North American society. Even the grandchildren of immigrants may lay claim to some home-country traditions of parents and grandparents. Yet there is a contradiction regarding how much the notion and reality of cultural diversity is really accepted. Some country-of-origin customs, such as food preparation, are well accepted by most Americans. Taco Bell is as American as McDonald's. Super Bowl commercials, which epitomize American pop culture, equally promote Pepsi, tacos, tortilla chips, and Budweiser beer as food for football fans. In contrast, the use of native languages and adherence to folk religion (both significant to cultural identity) are poorly tolerated. As a necessity, health institutions in the United States use Spanish when delivering services in locales with a high concentration of immigrant Latinos even though the popular use of foreign languages is rejected by most Americans. The English-only movement in the United States remains as strong today as when it was introduced in the 1980s (if not stronger), despite federal legislation supporting bilingual education.

In our view, ethnicity is the process through which some social groups are defined and define themselves. Ethnic identity is a personal attribute assigned to or chosen by individuals. Ethnic identity, as opposed to a set of cultural traditions, is not passed on from generation to generation but rather reinvented and reinterpreted by individuals in each generation.[25] It is, moreover, highly responsive to social and economic conditions and to how interethnic group relations at particular time periods are defined. This view emphasizes that ethnic identification is a creative process that evolves over time as the result of prolonged face-to-face contact between immigrants, their descendants, and their hosts.

Being Mexican American, for example, is not the same (even in a partial sense) as being an immigrant Mexican in the United States. Nor is being a Mexican American in one generation the same as being a Mexican American in another. In a popular 1970s play, *Zoot Suit,* there is a comic exchange between the protagonist, a teenage Latino boy, and his mother. The boy speaks in *pachuco* slang, to which his mother repeatedly objects. To the mother, the *pachuco* culture of East Los Angeles challenges and mocks the traditional Mexican culture in which she was raised and whose traditions she desperately attempts to have her son uphold.

Many immigrant parents work very hard to raise their children according to how they remember their own upbringing, actively attempting to slow down the Americanization process that molds their children in ways they do not approve. The outcome is often like that expressed by one Central American parent who was suddenly startled by an unexpected insight during a family therapy session. As her son's oppositional behavior and defiance in the face of her efforts to raise him like a good Guatemalan child were being addressed, she exclaimed: "I have never been more Guatemalan than after I came to the United States!" For children growing up in the United States, it is difficult enough to have their parents attempt to raise them within the traditions in which the parents were raised. It is almost intolerable to have their parents attempt to raise them according to an idealized cultural identity that does not even exist in the country of origin.

The following paragraphs describe Carlos, a second-generation Latino who spent much of his youth attempting to be "American." Now, as a parent who has found his Latino roots, he is trying to ensure that his children grow up with a strong Latino identity.

Carlos grew up in Los Angeles in a middle-class neighborhood. When he was a child, his mother scrubbed him with lemon on an *estropajo* (loofah) to lighten his skin color. As a teenager, he identified with the surfers for whom Los Angeles is well known. He dressed and played the part well; he listened to surfer music and spoke in surfer lingo. Then in college, he began to find his roots. He joined MEChA (Movimiento Estudiantil Chicano de Atzlán), changed his name from Charles to Carlos, began to listen to Mexican *rancheras,* and wore *guaraches* and Mexican peasant shirts.

Now married, Carlos brings to therapy his fifteen-year-old daughter Gabriela Mayahuel because she is rebellious and defiant at home. She loves "goth" and "darkwave" music, dresses in goth fashion, and hangs around a group that her father says is just "too strange and spooky." She has no Latino friends. In conversations with her father, she refuses to use the little Spanish that he taught her. Her middle name, her father tells the therapist, is the name of the Nahua goddess of the maguey plant, but everyone calls her Gabby. She angrily complains how, upon hearing her middle name, a student in her class recently started calling her Gabby Might-as-Well, which gave other students the impression that she was "easy." Naming her Gabriela was bad enough, she states, but calling her by a "stupid Aztec name" is unforgivable.

The dilemma that Carlos and his daughter experience illustrates how ethnic identity is relative to time, situation, and place. Its characteristics change over the course of an individual's life, as well as between generations, and are dependent on the particular cultural environments in which Latinos live.

Voluntary and Involuntary Immigration

The process of ethnicity is shaped by the history of a particular group. Some Latinos have come to the United States for economic opportunity and greater political freedom. Others are descendants of Latin Americans who were forced to become part of the United States by annexation or colonization. This distinction has been highlighted by Ogbu in his profile of *voluntary or immigrant minorities* and *involuntary minorities,* whose attitudes toward adaptation to the host culture differ.[26]

Voluntary groups willingly acquire selected aspects of North American culture because they do not view them as threatening to their cultural identity, which has been firmly established before immigration. Many Mexican immigrants to the Southwest are eager to learn English, often taking evening classes several nights a week even though they work full time.

In contrast, those whose ancestors were involuntarily incorporated into the United States often resist adopting certain values and attitudes as a way of differentiating themselves from the dominant culture. Despite extensive changes in their culture over the course of generations, they oppose complete assimilation, which is the essential process of the so-called melting pot. Although their culture has changed considerably from that of their ancestral heritage as a result of coping with and relating to the dominant group's culture, they invoke reconstructed versions of ancestral culture. They emphasize symbols, forms of behavior, or practices appropriate to themselves and different from those of the dominant culture. For these groups, there are dual frames of reference, one for the dominant culture and the other for their own group. A case in point is that of generations of New Mexican Latinos—involuntarily incorporated into the United States by the Treaty of Guadalupe Hidalgo in 1848—who have held on to some religious traditions, such as the Good Friday pilgrimage to the Sanctuario de Chimayó in New Mexico, the veneration of folk saints, and special rituals around the celebration of Christmas. A more unusual case is that of the descendants of the Crypto-Jews, or *Marranos,* in northern New Mexico, who officially converted to Catholicism during the Inquisition of the sixteenth century. These descendants unknowingly continue to practice rituals of Sephardic Jewish origin![27]

Among Latino groups, involuntary immigrants include some Mexican Americans and Puerto Ricans; voluntary immigrants include Mexicans, Cubans, Dominicans, and Central and South Americans. As already noted, Mexicans in the Southwest became part of the United States when the Texas territory was annexed as a result of the Treaty of Guadalupe Hidalgo. Puerto Ricans met the same fate following the Spanish-American War in 1898, at a time when they were just beginning to gain some autonomy from Spanish domination. Puerto Rico did not become self-governing until 1952 and is still considered to be a part of the United States, as a "free associated state." Therefore, all Puerto Ricans are citizens. This approach, which sees incorporation into U.S. society as voluntary or involuntary, also suggests that the meaning and impact of being bicultural or bilingual differ, for example, for Cubans (voluntary immigrants) and for some Mexican Americans (involuntary immigrants).

Other Sources of Variation

Besides this distinction between voluntary and involuntary status, there are other sources of variation within ethnic groups. For example, there are variations based on social class, physical characteristics (such as skin color), generational differences, urban versus rural origin, and legal versus illegal entry into the United States. Furthermore, poverty and education significantly shape ethnicity as a process. Last, geographic locales have important effects on between-group and within-group relationships and the ways in which immigrants adapt to the dominant culture.

An example of within-group differences can be found in Miami, which has the largest concentration of Cuban immigrants in the United States. The first waves of immigrants to Miami were white, urban, and from the upper and middle classes in Cuba. This wave gave rise to communities with strong political and economic bases and local cultures very similar to those of pre-Castro Cuba. These communities later were able to integrate subsequent waves of non-white, poor, and working-class Cuban immigrants and refugees.[28]

In contrast, Guatemalans as well as Salvadorans are more homogeneous with respect to lower social class, rural origin, and physical characteristics (dark skin and indigenous heritage). Often fleeing from political oppression and terror, severe economic scarcity, and violence arising from political movements (some backed by the United States), they are much more scattered throughout the United States and treated as economic burdens rather than political refugees. Each wave of immigrants continues to face unreceptive local communities, most of whom have little appreciation for the traumas these immigrants suffered in their countries and the survivors' guilt they often experience in regard to family members they have left behind.[29]

Cultural Diversity in the United States

If we are to take a contextual approach, we need a much broader view of the difficulties that Latino children and adolescents face. To understand the experience of Latinos in the United States, it is necessary to understand how the United States as a country has dealt with cultural diversity. A brief look at the history of immigration into the United States during the twentieth century reveals striking changes in how immigrants were received based on national policies and economic opportunities. This history is complicated by the changes in attitudes and policies toward Latino citizens, who were largely invisible in the United States until the civil rights movement became linked with the Mexican American and Puerto Rican nationalist movements in the 1960s.

The civil rights movement and the associated Latino nationalist movements emerged as the antithesis of assimilationist social ideologies and policies that dominated the first half of the twentieth century. The successive waves of largely European immigrants during the latter part of the nineteenth and early part of the twentieth centuries entered the United States at the height of the melting pot ideology. Translated into social programs, this ideology promoted the idea that the diverse cultures brought by the immigrants would mix and synthesize into a new and vigorous American culture.

The two world wars were a potent force in challenging the viability of this notion and underscored the national need to define Americans as not so different from their founding fathers, the Anglo-Americans. Thus, the Americanization process that resulted from the effects of the melting pot ideology became a process of imposed homogenization in which the rendered product looked and talked like Anglo-Americans.

At the same time, this process was being increasingly challenged by ethnic groups that were not so easily assimilated (the so-called unmeltable ethnics), either because of appearance (that is, race) and language or because they remained invisible in the American national image and silent in historical narratives. Puerto Ricans, as residents of the United States, are a good example. Few Americans are aware that Puerto Ricans—either on the continent or in Puerto Rico—are U.S. citizens with many of the rights thereof, including the freedom to move between the U.S. continent and Puerto Rico without restriction. Yet U.S.-based air carriers list San Juan, Puerto Rico, as an international destination, and residents of Puerto Rico do not have the full rights of U.S. citizens. According to the Jones Act of 1917, they cannot vote for the presidents who send them to war and they do not have representation in Congress. (In December 1998, Puerto Rico once again voted to maintain commonwealth status as a "free associated state" of the United States.) As another example, Mexican Americans have long endured the problems of being excluded from the American national image. Famous actors who began their careers before the revival of ethnic identities in the sixties—like Anthony Quinn, Rita Hayworth, Raquel Welch, and Martin Sheen—hid their ethnic identities to fit the American national image.

During the sixties, the presence of unmeltable ethnics such as Mexican Americans and Puerto Ricans was an attack on the melting pot ideology that had prevailed since the United States became a nation.[30] The unmeltable ethnics exhorted America to deny ethnicity no longer and to abandon the assimilation ideology that sought to erase cultural diversity from the American social panorama. However, the concept of unmeltable ethnics emphasizes continuity of cultural traditions over time, rather than the much more complex situation of a diversity of responses to being excluded from the American national image and from full participation in its rights and privileges.

Schwarz contrasts the official version of U.S. history as a pluralistic country that tolerates diversity and lives in multicultural harmony with its actual history, in which an American elite of Anglo-Saxon descent has consistently imposed its culture on ethnic minority groups. He states: "Thus, long before the United States's founding, and until probably the 1960s, the unity of the American people derived not from their warm welcoming of and accommodation to nationalist, ethnic, and linguistic differences but from the ability and willingness of an Anglo elite to stamp its image on other peoples coming to this country."[31]

In the United States, the term *ethnic* has come to apply only to those who are *not* white, middle-class, Anglo-Saxon, Protestant, or very similar to this type in appearance, social class, and behavior. As a result, the focus of ethnicity has shifted from cultural diversity to racial difference (such as the use of the term *people of color*) and political and economic disparity (such as the use of the term *ethnic minorities*). Despite decades of civil rights legislation, the social structure of the United States continues to be based on a racial order.[32]

Ironically, the response of the United States to the assertion of individual Latino identities by Chicanos and Puerto Ricans in the 1960s was to impose an ethnic-racial category—Hispanic—in which Latino cultural differences were homogenized. Now, rather than affirm authentic Latino identities derived from each national group's experience, Latinos must both "live up" to an idealized version of what it is to be "Hispanic" and battle among themselves for power and precedence regarding the benefits conferred by an imposed identity. In an anthropological study of ethnic labels and lives, Suzanne Oboler, a Peruvian American, cautions that "the new generations end up doing to themselves what the society has done to all Latinos: they homogenize, they stereotype, they categorize—and ultimately they divide themselves. They fracture the community. They break the self, not the mirror."[33]

Latino Social Traditions and Historical Contexts

All the Latino ethnic groups in the United States have traditions about social status from their countries of origin. In these countries, attitudes and values regarding external physical characteristics (skin color, hair form, and features), which are based on descent from colonized populations (Native American and African), are potent sources of negative, prejudicial feelings. Physical characteristics are aligned with socioeconomic status to create color and class hierarchies. In Mexico, Central America, and the Andean countries of South America, a majority of the population is *mestizo,* a mixture of Indian and European ancestries. Mestizos occupy a broad range of social class positions between an elite that traces its descent to Europe and the largely impoverished, indigenous peoples. In the Latin Caribbean (Cuba, Puerto Rico, and the Dominican Republic) and specific coastal regions of South America (for example, Colombia, Venezuela, and Ecuador) and Central America (for example, Panama, Nicaragua, Honduras, El Salvador, and Costa Rica), the lowest social stratum is occupied by persons of African descent. In countries that have both indigenous peoples and persons of African descent, the former are often socially marginalized, considered outside of national social classifications. As in other parts of Latin America, the elites in the Caribbean are, or appear to be, of European descent. A broad range of the color-class hierarchy between these two groups is occupied by people of mixed color (black and white), or *criollos.* There are exceptions to these social rules, as in Argentina, where groups of indigenous peoples and those of African descent are both small and marginalized and where those of European descent are socially and numerically dominant, eliminating the possibility of social mobility.

Where economic opportunities exist, peoples of color (mestizos, criollos, and indigenous Indians) can individually transcend the limitations imposed by color-class hierarchies by acquiring education and wealth. In the common parlance of some Latino countries, this is referred to as *blanquiarse* (to lighten oneself) or *levantarse* (to lift oneself up in the social hierarchy). Like the American elite of Anglo-Saxon descent in the United States, the Spanish elite of Latin America also consistently imposed its culture on ethnic minority groups. From the perspective of psychological treatment of Latino children and adolescents in the United States, what is important about these aspects of the history and social background of their Latino heritage is a legacy of discrimination. This legacy from their original countries lives on as a pervasive but unspoken theme among Latinos who have immigrated to the United States with the goal of attaining higher social status. It can become a potent source of unacknowledged conflict both within families and in interpersonal relationships. To complicate matters further, with immigration the effects of the legacy of discrimination are played out in another, perhaps even more difficult, environment of discrimination specific to the United States. The Garcias are a case in point.

The Garcias, Puerto Rican plantation laborers of mixed African and Spanish descent, are experiencing the discrimination often felt by immigrants. The Garcias saved their money for years in order to immigrate to Philadelphia, Pennsylvania. Mr. Garcia came first and worked at a cannery, which provided substandard group housing for male employees. Desiring an apartment in a neighborhood with good schools and few people of color (a measure of success in their country of origin), Mr. and Mrs. Garcia have been repeatedly turned away from homes in those neighborhoods without adequate explanation. Privately, Mr. Garcia expresses his frustration and anger that all of his efforts to *superar* (that is, transcend the color-class hierarchy of his country) have been futile. He struggles to understand the rejection he is encountering as a result of racism in the United States, which is based on the inheritance of physical characteristics.

Family and Community

The structure and organization of family life among Latinos originated in ancient agrarian societies typified by intensive small-plot horticulture. The indigenous peoples of Latin America lacked domestic animals as beasts of burden, and as a result land holdings and food production remained on a small scale and farm labor was limited to family members. Rural communities, in which the majority of the population lived, were small, composed of individuals related by kinship and marriage who developed complex cooperative networks. By the seventeenth century, large farms and ranches were established by the Spanish colonizers, who reorganized modes of production on a much larger scale, which required a community-based, as opposed to a family-based, labor force and was composed of native Indians at first and of mestizos later on.

In the eighteenth and nineteenth centuries in some tropical areas, the European elite established large plantations and international trade in food products (for example, coffee, chocolate, spices, tropical fruits). Lack of indigenous labor led them to import forced labor, largely from Africa, and establish new types of communities no longer based solely on kinship. Families, as corporate units of production, were no longer important in these areas. However, because laborers had to feed themselves, the small family plot remained essential, as did dependence on a nuclear family. Thus, the postconquest history of Latin America led to the centrality of two types of family life: the preferred form was the "extended family" made up of geographically close, cooperating relatives as independent farmers (the *campesinos,* or peasants); the other was the more isolated family unit with fewer ties to relatives and more ties to a class of workers with common interests (a proletarian class). The proletarian class supplied the first wave of migration to Latin American cities and later to the United States. As land became scarce because of redistribution in favor of the European elites and population growth, the *campesinos* also migrated to the cities.

The impact of this history is evident in present-day Latino family values of the importance of the extended family, and the family hierarchy, in which the oldest adult male dominates and in which position and power are structured according to age and gender. With immigration, the role of the extended family and its strong ethic of mutual obligations diminishes. The nuclear family becomes more important as a basic unit of survival, leading to an intensification of the preexisting, ideal pattern of interdependence among family members.

The relevance of changes in family organization can be appreciated in the case of Maria Elena and Juan, a Salvadoran couple who recently immigrated to the United States, leaving their three small children in the care of Maria Elena's parents. During the two years it took to earn enough money to bring over their children, they sent money to the grandparents that supported the entire household. Now that the children are reunited with their parents, Maria Elena expresses her intense guilt about no longer sending money to her parents, her overwhelming sense of burden in taking care of her three young children without her parents' help, and the need to be vigilant in the dangerous neighborhood in which they live. Her children complain that they feel too restricted, resent their parents' efforts to usurp the parental role of their grandparents, and express a great sense of loss of their grandparents.

Religion and Healing

All ethnic groups in the United States have brought with them their religious beliefs and practices, many of which are associated with healing. There is evidence that the practices have undergone significant changes over time, in part in response to the new cultural environment. As ethnic minority groups adapt to a difficult and often hostile society, and suffer considerable stress in the process, informal religious groups and individual religious healers, as well as the newer fundamentalist sects, take on even greater importance as ethnomedical healing systems, principally dealing with emotional distress and adjustment problems as well as the ubiquitous common maladies.[34] The healing rites are cultural expressions full of symbols with multiple meanings and represent concerns about ethnic identity, selfhood, family and community values, and affirmations of ethnic cohesiveness and traditions.

Latinos are mostly Catholic, although many have been converted to Protestantism, particularly Pentecostalism and similar fundamentalist sects. Some were converted before emigrating, and the process continues vigorously in the United States. In Latino communities, particularly among Puerto Ricans and Dominicans in the Eastern areas of the United States, *Espiritismo* (in some cases called *Espiritualismo*), a spirit-medium cult in which group healing sessions mediate between the sufferer and an envisioned world of various spirits of the dead, both intimate and famous, is widespread. *Santería* (or the *Lucumí* religion), an Afro-Cuban cult in which members individually or collectively worship syncretized representations of European saints and African gods with animal, plant, and money sacrifices, remains popular in Miami. These cults are based on popular (folk) Catholicism and are most often propagated through persons who are initiated when they undergo extreme suffering or near-death experiences. Santería was brought to Miami by Cubans, and it spread to the Northeast, Chicago, and even California during the seventies. Santería has now been syncretized with Espiritismo to produce still newer cults, such as *Mesa Blanca* in New York City.[35]

Curanderismo is the somewhat equivalent folk-healing system among Mexicans and Mexican Americans, although there is some debate about just how popular it is.[36] It differs from the Caribbean cults in that an individual practitioner is the main recourse for healing consultations. Curanderismo bases its practices on Catholic prayers and Native American and European herbal pharmacopeia. There is also a Mexican form of spiritualism in which the spirits who come to the sessions are usually folk saints. All of these healing cults are expressions of ethnic group autonomy in matters of health-seeking, particularly when biomedical healing fails or rejects a patient. They often operate in a complementary way to biomedicine, and they are widely reported to have beneficial psychological effects. Their persistence among some Latinos is testimony to the viability of Latino worldviews and self-views in which other than ordinary beings have a significant influence on human lives.

Although these forms of popular religion are found in all of the Latin American countries, they have somewhat different meanings for their communities of practitioners in the United States. Ana María Díaz-Stevens labels Latino popular religiosity as "communitarian spirituality."[37] She sees its most significant focus not as healing activity (in its broadest sense) but rather as building community. It is at one and the same time a protest against the hierarchies and power relationships integral to the established churches and resistance to being incorporated into an uncongenial spiritual community infused with unfamiliar customs and feelings.

Conclusion

In describing some of the main features of Latino cultures, we have attempted to illustrate how they vary. However, it is impossible to cover adequately the wide range of intra- and intercultural variation among Latinos in a single chapter. Despite this difficulty, we hope that the information we have provided will encourage practitioners to consider the complexities and richness of their clients' local worlds. In the chapters that follow, we further elaborate on how these cultural themes enter into the clinical arena.

Notes

1. L. Carroll, *Through the Looking Glass* (New York: St. Martin's Press, 1977), 36.
2. U. Bronfenbrenner, "Developmental Ecology Through Space and Time: A Future Perspective," in *Examining Lives in Context: Perspectives on the Ecology of Human Development,* ed. P. Moen, G. H. Elder Jr., and K. Lüscher (Washington, D.C.: American Psychological Association, 1995).
3. P. Cushman, "Ideology Obscured: Political Uses of the Self in Daniel Stern's Infant," *American Psychologist, 46* (1991): 206–219.
4. A. I. Hallowell, *Culture and Experience* (Philadelphia: University of Pennsylvania Press, 1955).
5. "The Story of César Chávez." [http://www.latinoweb.com/ufw/history.htm].
6. P. Dicochea and J. Mata, "Hispanic: What's in the Name?" (Hispanic Graduate Student Association of Arizona State University, Oct.-Nov. newsletter, 1997); R. Acuña, *Occupied America: A History of Chicanos* (New York: HarperCollins, 1988); G. Anzaldúa, *Borderlands = La Frontera: The New Mestiza* (San Francisco: Spinsters/Aunt Lute, 1987).
7. Dicochea and Mata, "Hispanic Graduate Student Association," p. 2.
8. U.S. Bureau of the Census, *Resident Population of the United States: Estimates by Sex, Race, and Hispanic Origin, with Median Age.* [http://www.census.gov/population/estimates/nation/intfile3–1.txt]. Dec. 28, 1998.
9. U.S. Bureau of the Census, *Hispanic Population Nears 30 Million,* Census Bureau Reports, Public Information Office, CB98–137. [http://www.census.gov/population/www/socdemo/hispanic.html]. Aug. 7, 1998.
10. U.S. Bureau of the Census, *Current Population Reports, Series P23–189, Population Profile of the United States: 1995* (Washington, D.C.: U.S. Government Printing Office, 1995).
11. U.S. Bureau of the Census, *Foreign-Born Population Reaches 25.8 Million, According to Census Bureau,* Public Information Office, CB98–57. [http://www.census.gov/population/www/socdemo/foreign.html]. Apr. 9, 1998.

12. U.S. Bureau of the Census, *Foreign-Born Population.*
13. U.S. Bureau of the Census, *Hispanic Population Nears 30 Million.*
14. U.S. Bureau of the Census, *Hispanic Population Nears 30 Million.*
15. U.S. Bureau of the Census, *Statistical Brief: The Nation's Hispanic Population, 1994,* SB/95–25 (Washington, D.C.: U.S. Department of Commerce, Economics and Statistics Administration, 1995).
16. U.S. Bureau of the Census, *Latino Americans Today* (Washington, D.C.: U.S. Government Printing Office, 1993).
17. U.S. Bureau of the Census, *Latino Americans Today.*
18. U.S. Bureau of the Census, *Statistical Brief.*
19. U.S. Bureau of the Census, *Latino Americans Today.*
20. U.S. Bureau of the Census, *Statistical Brief.*
21. U.S. Bureau of the Census, *Statistical Brief.*
22. U.S. Bureau of the Census, *California Leads States and Los Angeles County, Calif., Top Counties in Hispanic Population Increase,* Census Bureau Reports, Public Information Office, CB98–160. [http://www.census.gov/population/www/estimates/statepop.html].
23. U.S. Bureau of the Census, *California Leads States.*
24. F. Barth (ed.), *Ethnic Groups and Boundaries: The Social Organization of Cultural Difference* (Boston: Little, Brown, 1969).
25. M. J. Fischer, "Ethnicity and the Post-Modern Arts of Memory," in *Writing Culture,* ed. J. Clifford and G. E. Marcus (Berkeley: University of California Press, 1986), 194–233.
26. J. Ogbu, "From Cultural Differences to Differences in Cultural Frame of Reference," in *Cross-Cultural Roots of Minority Child Development,* ed. P. M. Greenfield and R. R. Cocking (Hillsdale, N.J.: Erlbaum, 1994), 365–391.
27. C. Pacheco and T. Atencio, "Manito Images and the Experience of Marginality: The Case of the Crypto-Jews and Genizaros," paper presented at the Sixth Annual Multicultural Mental Health Conference on Families and Children: When Cultures Connect—When Cultures Collide, Albuquerque, N.M. (May 14, 1992).
28. S. Oboler, *Ethnic Labels, Latino Lives: Identity and the Politics of (Re)Presentation in the United States* (Minneapolis: University of Minnesota Press, 1995).
29. A. M. Suarez-Orozco, *Central American Refugees and U.S. High Schools: A Psychosocial Study of Motivation and Achievement* (Stanford, Calif.: Stanford University Press, 1989).
30. W. Sollors, *Beyond Ethnicity: Consent and Descent in American Culture* (New York: Oxford University Press, 1986).
31. B. Schwarz, "The Diversity Myth: America's Leading Export," *Atlantic Monthly* (May 1995): 57–67.

32. Oboler, *Ethnic Labels.*
33. Oboler, *Ethnic Labels,* p. 173.
34. A. Harwood, *Rx: Spiritist as Needed* (New York: Wiley, 1977); J. D. Koss-Chioino, "Traditional and Folk Approaches Among Ethnic Minorities," in *Psychological Interventions and Cultural Diversity,* ed. J. F. Aponte, R. Y. Rivers, and J. Wohl (Needham Heights, Mass.: Allyn & Bacon, 1995), 145–163; S. J. Kunitz, *Disease, Change, and the Role of Medicine: The Navajo Experience* (Berkeley: University of California Press, 1983); R. Trotter and J. Chavira, *Curanderismo: Mexican Folk Healing* (Athens: University of Georgia Press, 1981).
35. V. Garrison, "The Puerto Rican Syndrome in Espiritismo," in *Case Studies in Spirit Possession,* ed. V. Crapanzano and V. Garrison (New York: Wiley, 1977), 383–450; Koss-Chioino, "Traditional and Folk Approaches."
36. M. J. Gilbert, "Mexican American Parents' Perceptions of Folk Childhood Disease: Little Evidence of a Strong Folk Tradition," paper presented at the annual meeting of the American Anthropological Association, Los Angeles (1980); M. Kay, "Health and Illness in a Mexican American Barrio," in *Ethnic Medicine in the Southwest,* ed. E. H. Spicer (Tucson: University of Arizona Press, 1977), 99–166; Trotter and Chavira, *Curanderismo.*
37. A. M. Díaz-Stevens, *Latino Popular Religiosity and Communitarian Spirituality,* Program for the Analysis of Religion Among Latinos (PARAL), Occasional Paper no. 4 (Sept. 1996).

Chapter Two

A Contextual Theory

With nothing to blame but the lack of contribution,
We gotta unite and utilize a solution.
PLACIDO VASQUEZ JR.

American psychology—particularly in this era of "empirically validated," "generalizable" treatments and "psychology as a science"—is experiencing challenges to its paradigms when they are applied to ethnic minorities in the United States as well as to other societies outside the United States. Despite these challenges, a recent American Psychological Association president was quoted as saying: "As we face managed care, it is my conviction that science is the bedrock on which practice rests and the best friend that practice has."[1] A growing number of books and articles are increasingly critical of basing psychology on an epistemology that reflects *only* the ethos of the society in which the epistemology has been developed—that is, the guiding beliefs of its people, groups, and institutions.[2] Moreover, Graham Richards draws attention to the fact that the concepts and practices of psychology are so much a part of the dominant culture that practitioners are unable to evaluate the ethical consequences of their practices.[3]

These challenges are illustrated in the case of Teresa, who receives inadequate and possibly inappropriate treatment.

Teresa, a fourteen-year-old Puerto Rican girl, is taken by her mother to see a psychologist through her health maintenance organization (HMO) because Mother is concerned about Teresa's periods of crying and overeating. The psychologist spends about fifteen minutes with Teresa while Mother anxiously sits in the waiting room. When the session ends, the psychologist informs Mother that her daughter is depressed, is most likely bulimic but appears to be hiding it, is a poor candidate for psychotherapy, and would benefit from a consult with a psychiatrist to determine if psychotropic medication might help. The psychologist is concerned about Teresa's unwillingness to talk to and confide in her. She further expresses concern to Mother about her overprotectiveness, Teresa's failure to establish age-appropriate independence, and Teresa's timidity and unassertiveness.

To the psychologist, Teresa is a depressed, passive-aggressive, possibly bulimic youngster who is psychologically crippled by illogical fears and anxieties. If Teresa were only more trusting and verbal, she would be an excellent candidate for cognitive behavioral therapy. But to her mother, Teresa is an unhappy adolescent who overeats when she is especially sad. Her mother recognizes that Teresa is intensely loyal to her because, as a single parent in the United States, she is trying to raise a proper Puerto Rican daughter and realistically worries about Teresa being negatively influenced by her peer group. However, Teresa sees herself as alienated from a peer group that has much more freedom than she has and is already sexually active. She appreciates her mother's desire to protect her and loves and respects her mother. As a compliant Puerto Rican teenager, she recognizes the importance of being deferential to persons in authority, such as the therapist. But she also finds it difficult to confide in such persons.

The services that Teresa received not only failed to address her problems in context but resulted in her being prescribed psychotropic medication, because the evaluation for treatment was individually focused. The psychologist did not attend to Teresa's relationship with her mother or to what Teresa and her mother considered to be appropriate behavior for her age and gender. This case illustrates how the psychologist neglected to consider the interaction among culture, development, and individual characteristics.

Universality and Interventions

In order to develop a contextual approach to psychological interventions for culturally diverse populations, we must first examine and describe the epistemology underlying the predominant forms of interventions in American psychology. Failure to do so may lead to the development of psychological interventions that are viewed as *culturally competent* from the dominant society's standpoint—

because they are based on the epistemology of that society—but that are not culturally responsive from the perspective of the ethnic minority population for which they are intended.

Two epistemologies have dominated American psychology: *positivism,* which treats human behavior as if it is a function of general laws independent of time and space, and *historicism,* which views human action as rooted in personal and evolutionary history.[4]

Positivism

According to James Faulconer and Richard Williams, positivism, with its faith in objectivity, detached observation, empiricism, logical positivism, and naive realism, has been the most influential psychological epistemology. Positivistic social science assumes that human behavior follows the model of the natural sciences and that it too can be understood and predicted by uncovering its hidden laws.

Historicism

Historicism entered the field of social science as a challenge to positivism. With regard to psychological interventions, historicism is exemplified by Freud's ideas and the psychoanalytic movement, which emphasize that early experiences of both individuals and the human species determine the structure of the psyche. Another widely used type of intervention, *behaviorism,* is a hybrid of positivism and historicism in that it objectifies personal history in terms of a reinforcement history or a process of socialization.[5]

Although psychological theories and practice based on these two epistemologies have made significant contributions, they also have certain limitations. First, the quest for universality inhibits a focus on culture.[6] The importance placed on experimental methodologies aimed at producing results that are replicable, generalizable, and lead to predictions of behavior, creates an implicit bias toward a search for universals. As a result, these theories fail to investigate and explain cultural differences based on relative values, meanings, and ideas. Second, the emphasis on objectivity—that is, the separation of the observer from the observed—leads to an artificial conversion of phenomena into objectified, measurable units (referred to as *variables*) that can be separated and analyzed apart from the phenomenon as experienced. Last, time is seen as a linear series of discrete and static events. A notion of causality is based on associations or relationships among these events. A corollary of this concept of causality is a focus on individuals as distinct from events and environmental elements. Thus, theories from these epistemologies cannot consider the "person participating in a sociocultural activity" as a unit of analysis or as a target for intervention.[7]

Contextualism as an Alternative

An alternative to theories based on positivism or historicism is *contextualism*. The notions of *context* and *situation* have been associated with a number of philosophers, including Karl Marx, John Dewey, and Stephen Pepper.[8] Prominent social scientists such as Lev S. Vygotsky, Roger Barker, Gregory Bateson, Urie Bronfenbrenner, and most recently Michael Cole have related contextualism to development.[9] According to Cole, developmental theories based on context can be divided into two types.[10] The first, which he labels "context as that which surrounds," views individual acts or events as embedded within a context that consists of all that an environment encompasses. Theories of this type, like Bronfenbrenner's ecological paradigm, emphasize levels of contexts and their interdependence. The second type, which Cole labels "context as that which weaves together," views context and the individual-in-action as intermeshed aspects of one biosocial, cultural process. Theories of this type, like those of Dewey, Pepper, and Vygotsky, focus on the interconnections between context and an event or activity.

Vygotsky regarded *activity* as an event within which the child, other persons, and the social-historical-cultural context are intermeshed; these three features make up a single unit or process.[11] Rather than identifying a particular stage that a child has reached and describing the characteristics exhibited by that child as evidence of development, Vygotsky advocated looking directly at the process of change. Both the child's context and the child must be studied. Contextualists recognize that developmental processes may differ across contexts.[12]

A Contextual Explanation of Cognitive Development

Vygotsky explains the process of cognitive development of the child-in-activity as mediated by psychological tools that include language, writing, maps, and other expressive media as well as technical tools that affect thinking, such as computers and calculators.[13] These tools can be thought of as products of a culture. Children use them to relate to their worlds; their use changes a person's thought processes. Tools on which high value is placed, and the social processes by which interchanges take place, are extremely variable across cultures and depend on the level of technological development in a particular society. For example, many American Indian parents teach by demonstration or modeling rather than through verbal or written instructions. Similarly, in a study of Mexican mothers in a small city, it was found that those who had little formal education taught by example, whereas those who had attended school were more likely to engage their children in verbal interaction. The children who attended secondary schools in this Mexican community were criticized by traditional parents as "complainers" who would rather talk than work, which indicated that the school experience reshaped communication patterns within the family.[14]

Cultural Practice

Many anthropologists who study development prefer the concept of *cultural practice* to that of activity, which is preferred by psychologists.[15] The notion of practice, which also weaves together development-in-context and the individual in a single process, goes further than the Vygotsky idea of activity. A cultural practice refers to recurring actions endowed with a meaning and a value that are shared with others in a particular context. Parents and teachers directing or controlling children represent kinds of cultural practices. Engaging in particular practices can lead to a sense of belonging and identity with a cultural group.

How Culture and Development Interrelate

An objectified focus on an individual child does not begin to account for the complex phenomena of child development or reflect developmental experiences from the child's viewpoint. Child development, as a process, can be thought of as culturally constructed not only through the settings or niches in which development takes place but also through complex interactions between development and culture.[16] In commenting on psychological studies of child development that take culture into account, Jan Valsiner notes that the approach of most developmental psychologists reduces culture to an independent variable, particularly in cross-cultural studies.[17] Comparisons across cultures are secondary in importance; the primary task should be to understand how cultures organize the conditions for development and how children react to them.[18] Contextual approaches to development strongly object to the notion that environment acts upon individuals. Proponents of these approaches advocate a paradigm that views the individual and his or her context as mutually active and reactive. Thus, both the child's developmental processes and her environmental niches can be said to co-create and reciprocally affect each other.

In the past, noncontextual theorists have described development as a series of tasks or stages that are programmed in concert with physiological changes throughout the life span. These were first seen as universally invariable. Although more recent studies consider individual variations in the timing of physical and physiological changes, relatively few examine how the nature of developmental tasks differs across cultures.[19] Significant questions have been raised regarding the relative contributions of nature (genes) versus nurture (environment).

Until recently, development was viewed as a fixed series of stages that people go through as they mature.[20] Jean Piaget proposed that there is a universal set of stages of cognitive development. Psychologists carrying out developmental research in other cultures found that the methods used to assess the stages were often unfamiliar and meaningless to children in non-European cultures. Therefore, the methods were useless in assessing cognitive development unless adapted to their cultural practices.[21] In a similar way, Sigmund Freud and Erik Erikson have come under criticism for proposing fixed stages of psychological and psychosocial development without explaining how the process of development unfolds or how their theories might be tested.[22] However, Erikson modified Freud's ideas in at least two important ways. He focused on social influences on development, an approach that he developed from experience in other cultures, and he added the important idea of identity as a primary goal of human life. These ideas suggested that the social environment affected development in a much more complex way than previously considered. The failure of stage theories to account adequately for the reciprocal relationship between the individual and the social environment has led to the greater acceptability of contextual theories of development.

A contextual approach to human development cannot overlook the reciprocal relationships between biology, psychology, and culture. It does not deny that there are universal aspects of development that include genetic programming, basic care of the dependent child, and socialization practices. These factors establish a general pattern for developmental change and interact with culture-specific factors. For example, everyone grows larger between infancy and adulthood. In a community in which cultural practices include having a competitive basketball program, a very tall and athletic teenager is not only highly esteemed but may also feel socially privileged. However, in many Latino cultures where soccer is the most popular sport, a very tall teenager may not only be at a disadvantage in this cultural practice but also feel socially handicapped. The interaction between universal aspects of development and cultural practices promotes continuity of culturally specific patterns across developmental stages.[23] It is unlikely that basketball will supplant soccer's popularity among immigrant Central American youth. However, as subsequent generations of Latino youth acquire height and participate in the cultural practices of North American society, their preference for sports may change. We take the position that development should be viewed as an integral part of the process of interactions between an individual and the many contexts in which transactions take place, including a biological-genetic dimension.

Contextual Approaches to Interventions

The concept of practice, defined by Sylvia Scribner and Michael Cole as "a recurrent goal-directed sequence of activities using a particular technology and particular systems of knowledge," fits well with classical notions of psychotherapy and other types of psychological interventions.[24] In therapy, the child or adolescent participates in two domains of cultural practices: those associated with a youth's development and the series of interchanges between the youth and the therapist. If we view therapy as addressing problems that emerge from relationships germane to child-rearing practices (such as those that include parents, peers, and teachers) and also focus on the child-therapist relationship, the practice of therapy and the practices of development merge as a single process.

When psychodynamic or behavioral therapists invoke the social environment as germane to an explanation of a client's problems, they are using context as an "add-on" to their basic view, which keeps the individual separate from his or her environmental niches.[25] In contrast, some contextualist practitioners view the world in terms of patterns of interactions between person and environment that cannot be understood by isolating the components (variables) of these interactions. Thus, they do not attempt to specify (and, in the case of behavioral or cognitive behavioral theorists, quantify) the unique contributions of these variables to explain a particular client's problem. For practitioners trained as positivists and historicists, thinking like a contextualist requires an abdication of the pervasive and intimate way that they have come to know "reality."

Currently, there are two main theories within contextualism in psychology that have given rise to clinical practice models: *developmental ecology* and *social constructivism*. Both theories have roots in such diverse fields as cultural anthropology; sociology; environmental, community, and developmental psychology; social ecology; ethology; and biological ecology.

Developmental Ecology

The general premise of ecologically oriented therapies is that problems arise because of lack of *environmental fit* between the individual and the environment.[26] As Richard Munger explains: "A clinician must identify the variables in the environment that affect the child's conduct. Settings must be defined that will spur the child toward the specific changes desired. Finally, decisions must be made about selecting, changing, and creating settings to address the child's behavior."[27]

Ecologically oriented practitioners view assessment as a process of systematically organizing the steps necessary to change the ecosystem so that it functions optimally for an individual.

Social Constructionism

Following anthropologists like A. I. Hallowell, whom we mentioned in Chapter One, social constructionists view an individual's reality as culturally constructed. One of their main premises is that "beliefs, values, institutions, customs, labels, laws, divisions of labor, and the like that make up our social realities are constructed by the members of a culture as they interact with one another from generation to generation and from day to day. That is, societies construct the 'lenses' through which their members interpret their world. The realities that each of us take for granted are the realities that our societies have surrounded us with since birth."[28]

From a social constructionist perspective, the therapist-client relationship is a partnership aimed at assisting the client to create a new reality. In order to solve problems or deal with emotional distress, social constructionist practitioners, although acknowledging the influence of the past, focus on the resources and strengths of the client toward reconstructing a more positive future life.[29]

In ecological models, the individual (with his or her biological and psychological endowment) is seen as being in active interaction with the external environment, each changing and affecting the other. Both social constructionism and narrative therapies are based on what William J. Lyddon calls *formal contructivism*, which is a contextual worldview.[30] Formal constructivism "emphasizes the inseparable connection among psychological (personally constructed), contextual (socially constructed), and temporal dimensions of experience."[31]

In developing our approach to working with Latino youth in ways that are culturally and developmentally responsive, we have integrated aspects of the social constructionist perspective into a developmental ecological framework. Furthermore, our clinical method borrows aspects of the ethnographic approach in anthropology. In the sections that follow, we describe the elements we have borrowed from these three sources.

Developmental Ecology as a Basis for Interventions

In his earlier work, Bronfenbrenner proposed that *context* (environment or situation) is composed of four interrelated levels:

- The *microsystem* consists of face-to-face settings in which a particular individual is involved (for example, family, school, peer group).
- The *mesosystem* includes two or more linked settings that include the individual (for example, school-family).
- The *exosystem* is made up of linkages between two or more settings, only one of which includes the individual (for example, street gang and his or her mother's *comadres*).
- The *macrosystem* overarches all of the other systems in a particular culture, subculture, or larger context. It serves as a template that defines general cultural patterns. These patterns may be stylistic (for example, gang members in California and Massachusetts dress and act similarly), moral (for example, a belief that sexual activity should not occur among adolescents), political (for example, a belief that an individual has a right to bear arms), socioeconomic (for example, level of income determines lifestyle), and ideological (for example, individuals who are psychologically healthy have a sense of self that is masterful and independent).[32]

In his more recently described bioecological paradigm, Bronfenbrenner expands his theory of ecological systems in several ways. First, he gives greater emphasis to the importance of enduring forms of interactions that he calls *proximal processes,* such as child-parent or child-child interactions. Second, he adds the component of historical time to the notion of environment. That is, a person's life course is patterned by particular circumstances and situations in the historic period in which he or she lives. This influences each generation's ideas of how to rear its children. For example, today's socialization of girls is shaped by the prominence of feminism as an ideal that promotes equality with boys. Third, he incorporates the biological domain, much as we have described earlier in this chapter. Fourth, he highlights the interaction among the "active, evolving, biopsychological individual," which includes the notion of life span and developmental timing, proximal processes, immediate and remote environments (context), and historical events.[33] Bronfenbrenner's new model is a temporalized, contextual one that is compatible with Vygotsky's notion of activity and Cole's notion of practice.[34] In his expanded model, Bronfenbrenner moves away from a notion of context as that which surrounds and moves toward a formulation of context as that which weaves together.

Our Approach to Interventions

We feel that Bronfenbrenner's expanded model is very suitable as a template for conceptualizing and developing culturally and developmentally responsive psychological interventions.[35] In adapting his model to interventions that incorporate selected aspects of the social constructivist perspective and contributions from the ethnographic method in anthropology, we emphasize the following:

- *Contexts must be viewed as interwoven in order to avoid the risk that a particular level be considered as temporally or causally more important.* A child with a history of seizure disorder who has severe explosive outbursts associated with these seizures may be treated solely with anticonvulsants. However, the severe explosive outbursts may be equally associated with family interactions and dynamics.
- *The notion of interwoven contexts avoids the tendency for concepts based on nested contexts to ignore the dynamic relationships between levels, thereby treating the contexts as either stimuli or causes.*[36] In the case of the child with seizure disorder, there might be a strong temptation to view his seizures, and the apparently concomitant explosive episodes, as solely or primarily biological in nature, and thus neglect potential interventions that address the family dynamics. The child's behavior must be understood as influenced by different dimensions of his environment in relationship to his internal states and characteristics that include his neurophysiology, cognitions, expectations, attributions, and motivations.
- *We must take culture into account as the symbolic system that underlies behavior when we intervene in a youth's environment.* As Jerome Bruner notes regarding the way psychologists have overlooked culture in treating clients: "The symbolic systems that individuals used in constructing meaning were systems that were already in place, already 'there,' deeply entrenched in culture and language."[37] In order to avoid what we described as the Red Queen phenomenon in Chapter One, the practitioner must come to understand the youth's search for meaning in relation to his or her local worlds. In this effort, practitioners must also understand their own cultural

worlds and how those worlds affect the relationship with the youth, including the goals for therapy and the practitioner's expectations of the youth.

• *We need to consider the influences of both personal and cultural history that mediate changes across generations.* In Chapter One, we described how César Chávez may have been shaped by the circumstances of both his personal and his cultural history—his moment in time and place. Our use of historical time is not intended to provide a causal explanation for behavior; rather, it provides the basis for interpreting a youth's behavior in the here and now as situated within a cultural context, rich in history and tradition.

• *We must address aspects central to dealing with culturally diverse youth.* These include markers of social position (race, skin color, social class, ethnicity, and gender), mechanisms of social stratification (racism, prejudice, discrimination, and oppression), types of segregation (residential, economic, social, and psychological), processes of culture change (immigration and acculturation), and types of positive and negative environments (schools, health care systems, and juvenile justice systems).[38]

• *Ethnography is a useful method for acquiring knowledge about the youth's local worlds, both the environments in which the youth interacts and the cultural contexts that provide meanings for those actions.* Ethnography is a method of inquiry that charts and describes environment, behavior, and relationships—all that is constituted by a local world.[39] In anthropology, it is often referred to as *fieldwork.* Ethnography focuses on how people in worlds unfamiliar to the ethnographer represent and interpret their worlds. It is an interactive and collaborative process in which the ethnographer becomes part of the situation being studied, yet remains separate enough to describe the patterns and range of variation within the culture. The ethnographer enters the field of study with respect for the participants and humility about how little he or she knows about them. In our approach, the practitioner employs an ethnographic process of inquiry in order to understand the relevant meanings in context necessary to assess the youth's "problem" and formulate a culturally and developmentally responsive intervention.[40]

• *Each dimension of the bioecological paradigm (process-person-context-time) is framed by culture, promoting cultural responsiveness for all types of interventions.* For example, the proximal process of child-parent interactions is culturally patterned by particular values (*respeto,* respect, and *humilidad,* humility) and ideas (girls must be protected, whereas boys are given much more freedom in early adolescence). Or in the late 1990s Latino youth may no longer benefit from affirmative action in the same way that their parents may have in the 1970s.

- *In our contextual approach, particular therapeutic techniques, such as those used in behavioral, cognitive-behavioral, family, and narrative therapies, can be used in the large complex of contextually based interventions.* The point here is that, if compatible with the youth's and family's goals, ideas, and motivations, a diverse set of therapeutic techniques can be used within a contextual formulation that is culturally and developmentally responsive without committing to the theories underlying specific techniques.

Assessment from a Contextual Framework

In our approach, clients are not viewed as separate from their environments, whether these are families, peers, schools, neighborhoods, church groups, or larger communities that include the national society. Contextual therapists recognize that the interrelationships between Latino youth and their environments are bidirectional and interactive rather than unidirectional and additive, which is often an assumption in therapies based on behavioral, cognitive-behavioral, psychodynamic, and medical models. For example, we would *not* say that Carlos, a boy of fourteen, becomes sad, despondent, and suicidal because he has developed a clinical depression as a result of an inherent vulnerability or identified stressful life events. Neither would we investigate the problem of depression in the youth by identifying and assessing the discrete and unidirectional effects of variables such as school failure, rejection by peers, or family dysfunction. Instead, we would examine and describe interactions between Carlos and the environments in which he participates—for example, the interactions between Carlos and his family, his peers, his teachers, his ethnic community, and the larger society in which he lives.

In our clinical approach, we describe how individuals and environments interrelate. For instance, instead of talking about a substance-abusing adolescent or attributing the problem to a diagnostic category, we would describe the situations in which an adolescent uses substances. We would ask the following questions: What are the attitudes of his family members toward substance use? Do his parents or other family members use or abuse substances? Does the family support activities (such as church participation, parental monitoring, family recreational activities) that would inhibit or protect against the use of substances? Does he have a group of friends who use or do not use drugs? Under what conditions (for example, alone, at parties, as part of gang activities) does he use drugs? Is he successful academically and socially in school? Are his parents involved in the school he attends? Does he live in poverty or in a densely populated neighborhood in which drug dealing is common? Has he been abused or otherwise traumatized early in life? Has he been the object of discrimination in the community or at school? This process of inquiry into environmental contexts elucidates the transactional nature of the person-environment contexts involved in this adolescent's substance use.

An Illustration of Our Contextual Model: Hugo

As an example of interwoven contexts, we might consider the case of Hugo, a sixteen-year-old Mexican boy who has resided in California for the past three years with his father and mother, both migrant laborers. Hugo's two younger siblings are living in Mexico with their paternal grandparents. Hugo is torn between helping his parents in the fields to earn more money to bring his siblings to the United States and wishing to spend time with his nonmigrant classmates. His best friends, none of whom are involved with gangs or any delinquent activities, have interests in many more leisure activities than were available to Hugo when he was in Mexico (for example, skateboarding, surfing, going to rock concerts). He is very popular with both boys and girls. His teachers see him as an exceptional teenager who has avoided the pitfalls that other children of migrant parents have succumbed to. At a recent parent night, several of his teachers told his parents that he was a great role model for his peers.

Hugo has a Vietnamese girlfriend whom he regularly meets at the shopping mall. His parents express concern because she is neither Christian nor Latina. Her parents, who speak mostly Vietnamese, are equally concerned about Hugo's different race and religion and do not feel they know him well enough to trust him.

For Hugo, some of the *microsystems* are (1) Hugo and his parents; (2) Hugo and his teachers; (3) Hugo and his girlfriend; and (4) Hugo and the gang members. Some of the *mesosystems* consist of (1) Hugo's parents and his teachers; (2) Hugo's own family and his girlfriend's family; and (3) Hugo's friends and his girlfriend. Two examples of *exosystems* are (1) Hugo's father's company and Hugo's family; and (2) Hugo's girlfriend's family and their Buddhist temple community. At least three *macrosystems* can also be identified: (1) the U.S. culture, which sets standards for Hugo's school experience, leisure activities, lifestyle, and so on; (2) the Mexican culture, which sets expectations regarding adolescent sexuality, relationship with parents (conceptualized as *respeto*), spirituality, and work obligations to the family; and (3) the Vietnamese culture, which also sets expectations regarding adolescent sexuality and proper marriage partners, relationship with parents (conceptualized as filial piety), and religious obligations.

From a description of Hugo's activities and cultural practices across these levels of context, we can attempt to understand Hugo's behavior. We can understand how Hugo's activities take on meanings as they are interwoven into a much larger life tapestry. Image the following scenario: Hugo gets his girlfriend pregnant, upsetting both sets of parents and creating intense conflict among all members of both families. He wants to drop out of school in order to get a job as a farm laborer, a job he had previously said he would never want. When a teacher with whom he has been very close tries to convince him to stay in school, Hugo reacts in a defiant and angry manner, much to his teacher's surprise. From the perspective of a contextual model, we might suggest that Hugo has become overwhelmed by the ideal that others have for him. Despite encouragement from his parents and teachers, Hugo has strong doubts about achieving the moral and educational ideals that others have proposed for him. He takes recourse in a traditional practice of young fatherhood—much like his father did before him. His previous effort to find acceptance outside of his own ethnic group has been suddenly preempted by the potent influences of Mexican gender ideals and ethnic identity to which his upbringing has exposed him. The defiance he expresses to his teacher might be understood in part as emanating from his sense that he is being asked to abdicate a valued cultural role (being a responsible father and caring partner). Thus, a contextual approach to psychological intervention would address all of these levels of context to arrive at an effective solution.

Conclusion and Organization of Following Chapters

This chapter has described the four contextual levels; these levels are used to organize the chapters that follow. It should be noted, however, that we use these levels to focus on areas for assessment and intervention without assuming that each one represents a discrete context. Each level can be thought of as a different view on the interplay of proximal processes, the developing individual (which includes the life span from infancy to adulthood), and historical time (events that occur in the more remote environments in an individual's life, and events that go across generations). Focusing on these contextual levels is akin to shining a flashlight with a progressively widening beam on an area of interest.

In Chapters Five, Seven, and Eight, we focus on mesosystems, exosystems, and macrosystems, respectively, and their interplay with process, person, and time. At each of these levels, both the contexts and dimension of time broadens. In the macrosystem, which is the broadest context of cultural practices (similar to Vygotsky's notion of activity), traditions are transmitted from generation to generation with varying degrees of continuity. For example, the Spanish language has been passed on to many cultures and despite generational and regional differences, a Spanish-speaking person from Guatemala in the twentieth century can understand eighteenth-century Castilian Spanish. In contrast, the Catholicism practiced in Spain in the sixteenth century has been syncretized with Native American religious beliefs, as illustrated by *La Virgen de Guadalupe* in Mexico.

But first, in Chapter Three, we turn to microsystems, examining face-to-face interactions with persons, objects (similar to Vygotsky's psychological tools), and symbols (such as ideals and language), as Bronfenbrenner has recently described. The microsystem, which is the narrowest context, includes processes—such as mother-child relationships, determining where the child sleeps, or types of discipline.

Notes

1. S. Sleek, "The 'Cherrypicking' of Treatment Research," *American Psychological Association Monitor* (Dec. 1997): 1.

2. J. E. Faulconer and R. N. Williams, "Temporality in Human Action: An Alternative to Positivism and Historicism," *American Psychologist, 40*(11) (1985): 1179–1188; *Critical Psychology: An Introduction,* ed. D. Fox and I. Prilleltensky (London: Sage, 1997); H. Landrine, "Clinical Implications of Cultural Differences: The Referential Versus the Indexical Self," *Clinical Psychology Review, 12*(4) (1992): 401–415; G. Richards, *Putting Psychology in Its Place: An Introduction from a Critical Historical Perspective* (New York: Routledge, 1996); E. E. Sampson, "The Debate on Individualism: Indigenous Psychologies of the Individual and Their Role in Personal and Societal Functioning," *American Psychologist, 43*(1) (1988): 15–22; J. Bruner, *Acts of Meaning* (Cambridge, Mass.: Harvard University Press, 1990).

3. Richards, *Putting Psychology in Its Place.*

4. Faulconer and Williams, "Temporality in Human Action."

5. Faulconer and Williams, "Temporality in Human Action."

6. This critique is in direct contrast to that of H. Betancourt and S. R. Lopez, "The Study of Culture, Ethnicity, and Race in American Psychology," *American Psychologist, 48*(6) (1993), who assert that "the main limitation of mainstream theories is that they ignore culture and therefore lack universality" (p. 634).

7. P. J. Miller and J. J. Goodnow, "Cultural Practices: Toward an Integration of Culture and Development," in *Cultural Practices as Contexts for Development,* ed. J. J. Goodnow, P. J. Miller, and F. Kessel, New Directions for Child Development, no. 67 (San Francisco: Jossey-Bass, 1995), 5–16.

8. M. Cole, "The Supra-Individual Envelope of Development: Activity and Practice, Situation and Context," in *Cultural Practices as Contexts for Development,* ed. J. J. Goodnow, P. J. Miller, and F. Kessel, New Directions for Child Development, no. 67 (San Francisco: Jossey-Bass, 1995); K. Marx, "Theses on Feuerbach," in *Writings of the Young Marx on Philosophy and Society,* ed. L. D. Easton and K. H. Guddat (New York: Doubleday, 1967 [Originally published 1845]); J. Dewey, *Logic: The Theory of Inquiry* (Austin, Tex.: Holt, Rinehart and Winston, 1938); S. Pepper, *World Hypotheses* (Berkeley: University of California Press, 1942).

9. R. G. Barker, *Ecological Psychology: Concepts and Methods for Studying the Environment of Human Behavior* (Stanford, Calif.: Stanford University

Press, 1968); G. Bateson, *Steps to an Ecology of Mind* (New York: Ballantine, 1972); L. S. Vygotsky, "The Instrumental Method in Psychology," in *The Concept of Activity in Soviet Psychology*, ed. J. V. Wertsch (Armonk, N.Y.: Sharpe, 1981). Pepper's treatise on world hypotheses and Vygotsky's theories have especially inspired studies of development based on the notion of context.

10. Cole, "The Supra-Individual Envelope."

11. An overview of Vygotsky's theories is provided in M. Cole, "Culture and Development," in *Developmental Psychology: An Advanced Textbook*, 3rd ed., ed. M. Bornstein and M. Lamb (Hillsdale, N.J.: Erlbaum, 1992); P. H. Miller, *Theories of Developmental Psychology* (New York: Freeman, 1993); R. Van der Veer and J. Valsiner, *Understanding Vygotsky: A Quest for Synthesis* (Oxford, England: Blackwell, 1991); *Context and Development*, ed. R. Cohen and A. W. Siegel (Hillsdale, N.J.: Erlbaum, 1991).

12. Miller, *Theories of Developmental Psychology*.

13. Vygotsky, "The Instrumental Method"; Miller, *Theories of Developmental Psychology*.

14. F. M. Tapia Uribe, R. A. LeVine, and S. E. LeVine, "Maternal Education and Maternal Behaviour in Mexico: Implications for the Changing Characteristics of Mexican Immigrants to the United States," *International Journal of Behavioral Development*, *16*(3) (special issue, 1993): 395–408.

15. Miller and Goodnow, "Cultural Practices." The idea of practice is taken from the work of P. Bourdieu, *Outline of a Theory of Practice* (New York: Cambridge University Press, 1977).

16. S. Harkness and C. M. Super, "The Cultural Construction of Child Development: A Framework for the Socialization of Affect," *Ethos*, *11*(4) (1983): 221–231.

17. J. Valsiner, *Human Development and Culture* (Lexington, Mass.: Heath, 1989).

18. Valsiner, *Human Development and Culture*.

19. See, however, M. Cole, "Cross-Cultural Research in the Sociohistorical Tradition," *Human Development*, *31* (1988): 137–157; "Context, Modularity, and the Cultural Constitution of Development," in *Children's Development Within Social Context*, vol. 2, *Research and Methodology*, ed. L. T. Winegar and J. Valsiner (Hillsdale, N.J.: Erlbaum, 1992); M. Cole, J. Gay, J. A. Glick, and D. W. Sharp, *The Cultural Context of Learning and Thinking* (New York: Basic Books, 1971); P. M. Greenfield and C. P. Childs, "Developmental Continuity in Biocultural Context," in *Context and Development*, ed. R. Cohen and A. W. Siegel (Hillsdale, N.J.: Erlbaum, 1991).

20. Greenfield and Childs, "Developmental Continuity," p. 136.

21. M. Cole and S. Scribner, *Culture and Thought: A Psychological Introduction* (New York: Wiley, 1974).
22. Miller, *Theories of Developmental Psychology;* J. L. Briggs, "Mazes of Meaning: How a Child and a Culture Create Each Other," in *Interpretive Approaches to Children's Socialization,* ed. W. A. Corsaro and P. J. Miller, New Directions for Child Development, no. 58 (San Francisco: Jossey-Bass, 1992), 25–49.
23. Greenfield and Childs, "Developmental Continuity."
24. S. Scribner and M. Cole, *The Psychology of Literacy* (Cambridge, Mass.: Harvard University Press, 1981), 235.
25. J. Valsiner and L. T. Winegar, "Contextualizing Context: Analysis of Metadata and Some Further Elaborations," in *Children's Development Within Social Context,* vol. 2, *Research and Methodology,* ed. L. T. Winegar and J. Valsiner (Hillsdale, N.J.: Erlbaum, 1992).
26. R. L. Munger, "Ecological Trajectories in Child Mental Health," in *Innovative Approaches for Difficult-to-Treat Populations,* ed. S. W. Henggeler and A. B. Santos (Washington, D.C.: American Psychiatric Press, 1997).
27. Munger, "Ecological Trajectories," p. 13.
28. J. Freedman and G. Combs, *Narrative Therapy: The Social Construction of Preferred Realities* (New York: Norton, 1996), 16.
29. M. F. Hoyt, "Introduction: Competency-Based Future-Oriented Therapy," in *Constructive Therapies,* ed. M. F. Hoyt (New York: Guilford Press, 1994).
30. W. J. Lyddon, "Forms and Facets of Constructivist Psychology," in *Constructivism in Psychotherapy,* ed. R. A. Neimeyer and M. J. Mahoney (Washington, D.C.: American Psychological Association, 1995).
31. Lyddon, "Forms and Facets," p. 78.
32. U. Bronfenbrenner, "Ecological Systems Theory," *Annals of Child Development,* vol. 6, *Six Theories of Child Development,* ed. R. Vasta (Greenwich, Conn.: JAI Press, 1989).
33. U. Bronfenbrenner, "Developmental Ecology Through Space and Time: A Future Perspective," in *Examining Lives in Context: Perspectives on the Ecology of Human Development,* ed. P. Moen, G. H. Elder Jr., and K. Lüscher (Washington, D.C.: American Psychological Association, 1995).
34. Bronfenbrenner, "Developmental Ecology."
35. J. Szapocznik, M. A. Scopetta, A. Ceballos, and D. Santisteban, "Understanding, Supporting, and Empowering Families: From Microanalysis to Macrointervention," *The Family Psychologist, 10*(2) (1994): 23–27. The authors use Bronfenbrenner's earlier ecological model to describe how they developed psychological interventions within each of these systems.

36. Cole, "The Supra-Individual Envelope."

37. J. Bruner, *Acts of Meaning* (Cambridge, Mass.: Harvard University Press, 1990), 11.

38. C. Garcia Coll and others, "An Integrative Model for the Study of Developmental Competencies in Minority Children," *Child Development, 67* (1996): 1891–1914.

39. *Handbook in Cultural Anthropology,* ed. R. Bernard (Walnut Creek, Calif.: Altamira Press, 1998).

40. For a discussion of the clinician as ethnographer, see E. B. Brody, "The Clinician as Ethnographer: A Psychoanalytic Perspective on the Epistemology of Fieldwork," *Culture, Medicine, and Psychiatry, 5* (1981): 273–301.

Chapter Three

Latino Youth in Personal Contexts

My appearance is sloppy, my home's a jalopy,
A positive role model, there's no one to copy.
PLACIDO VASQUEZ JR.

Latino youths live in many worlds, each delimited by particular patterns of family, peer, and school relationships. Consider the case of Beto, by all accounts a very talented, bright, and popular high school junior. His teachers see him as becoming a sure success at one of the prestigious colleges that are actively recruiting him. Beto is the oldest of five children in a family abandoned by the father. Despite many struggles, his mother has managed to keep the children in school and out of trouble. All five children are very good students, well liked by both peers and teachers.

When Beto declines a number of university scholarships and decides to attend community college instead, his teachers are dismayed and his non-Latino classmates shocked. Advice given by teachers and guidance counselor has no effect on changing Beto's mind. At home, Beto is a loyal and exemplary son who is dutifully complying with his mother's expectations that he help her raise his siblings. Although Beto is somewhat disappointed, he feels a strong sense of honor and self-respect associated with his decision to stay at home. But to the teachers who have worked hard to help him achieve his potential, Beto's choice represents flawed judgment that will doom him to career failure. Was Beto's decision right or wrong? How can we better understand how and why Beto made his decision?

In this chapter, we explore relationships within the immediate environments—or microsystems—in which Latino youth live. We first consider the *biopsychological characteristics* (that is, the expression of their genetic inheritance, both physically and psychologically, and developmental events such as traumas and illnesses) with which Latino youths present at a given time in interaction with persons, objects, and symbols in their immediate environment.[1] As we described in Chapter Two, proximal processes are influenced by immediate and remote environments and by personal and cultural history.[2]

We then explore relationships in immediate face-to-face settings between an individual and family, school, and peers. Because our description of proximal processes is intended to demonstrate a contextual approach to formulating interventions, we briefly discuss the patterning of proximal processes for Latino youth in two areas of activity: parenting and spirituality. Next, we discuss the role of language, sense of self, and ethnic and racial socialization at this level of analysis, because we believe these aspects are central to conducting culturally responsive interventions and to understanding development in context. Finally, we discuss the limitations of noncontextual models of psychopathology and recent trends toward contextualizing diagnosis in response to these limitations.

The Maturing Biopsychological Individual

The biopsychological characteristics of an individual are defined according to the time in which they occurred, and they range from cognitive and language abilities to brain impairment and illnesses like diabetes or asthma. From a contextual perspective, an individual is not simply born with innate abilities or attributes; instead, proximal processes shape the developing individual. Helen Keller is an example of an individual who rises above the limitations of her biopsychological endowment as a result of the proximal processes she experienced. With the help of a gifted and dedicated teacher, she learned to read using the Braille system, to write using a specially constructed typewriter, and later to speak. She subsequently attended Radcliffe College and became a renowned author and lecturer. In Chapter One, we suggested how the life of César Chávez was similarly influenced by interactions with his parents, that is, by one kind of proximal process.

We conceptualize time, that is, the temporal aspect of development, in two ways. The first refers to the course of time that elapses as the individual grows. Time in this sense is thought of as the biological consequences of maturation. A brain injury that is not immediately treated may have different consequences than would the same injury if treated immediately. A man in his seventies can no longer play sports or learn as well as he did when he was twenty-five. The second conceptualization of time refers to historical, transgenerational time, without its biological implications—in other words, to cultural history. A person who was a child during World War II has had very different experiences than a child growing up today.

In this section, we focus on time in the maturational sense as it affects the biopsychological individual. The maturational history of a child can inform us about how biopsychological characteristics influence the patterning of proximal processes like parent-child interactions. The following case illustrates how a biopsychological characteristic—a seizure disorder that was not recognized as influencing behavior—contributed to the development of severe behavioral and emotional problems in a Latino boy. In this case, failure to attend to the seizure disorder led to attributing the problems to other proximal processes, such as parent-child interactions.

Pepe, a ten-year-old Salvadoran boy, is admitted to a psychiatric hospital because of temper outbursts, which have become very frequent, intense, and prolonged. Pepe's temper outbursts last as long as an hour and a half three times a day. He has to be physically restrained to prevent him from hurting others and destroying property. His parents are desperate for help in managing his behavior. He has been seen by a number of providers who told his parents that his problems are caused by behavioral disorders that include conduct disorder, attention-deficit hyperactivity disorder, and intermittent explosive disorder, and by a variety of psychosocial and psychocultural factors. Attributing his problems to psychosocial factors, such as that Pepe was the product of a rape by a neighbor (a "secret" that had been kept from Pepe and his siblings) and to psychocultural factors, such as acculturative stress and indigenous beliefs of the mother about the meaning of the rape and birth, have left his mother overwhelmed with guilt and shame. His stepfather, whom Pepe and his siblings believe to be Pepe's biological father, experiences much guilt and confusion about the complicity with his wife regarding Pepe's birth father. For them, Pepe's problems are the result of "parenting out of deception," of the evil Pepe carries within him from his birth father, and of the sins his parents had committed. The diagnoses (conduct disorder, attention-deficit hyperactivity disorder, and intermittent explosive disorder), which implicate biopsychological processes within Pepe himself and do not clarify the etiology of the problems, have done little to help them deal with his problems.

During the administration of a continuous performance test (a computerized vigilance test used as part of an assessment of attentional processes), the newly assigned clinician notices that Pepe loses track of what he is seeing on the computer monitor for short spans of time. During these episodes, he moves his mouth in a curious manner. When the clinician asks his parents if they had noticed this behavior at home, his mother states that they noticed this long before and even had a nickname for him (*El Sapito*, the little frog) because of the way he moves his mouth. The clinician requests a neurological evaluation, suspecting that Pepe might have a seizure disorder. It is soon established that Pepe suffers from partial complex and absence seizures. The mother's pregnancy with Pepe had been very difficult and she had been very depressed throughout the pregnancy. Labor had been long. Pepe was born prematurely and his birth weight was very low. His motor development appeared advanced but his language development had been delayed. A subsequent neuropsychological evaluation reveals significant receptive and expressive language and other processing problems. Although Pepe's behavioral problems stem from multiple causes, a trial of valproic acid does much to reduce the intensity, frequency, and length of his temper outbursts. Furthermore, greater specification of his neurocognitive deficits allows the hospital staff to design a school and milieu program that gives him a greater sense of competence and decreases the intense frustration he feels when asked to perform in the areas of greatest deficit. Likewise, his parents are instructed on ways to work more effectively with his neurocognitive deficits, which not only benefits Pepe but gives them a new sense of efficacy and a renewed sense of hope.

The case of Pepe shows the interaction between biopsychological characteristics and proximal processes. It also highlights how this interaction is essential to an adequate appraisal of a youth's problems.

We should mention that the innate difference model, which is still evident in mental health practice, looks at the biopsychological individual without much, if any, attention to either context or proximal processes. In the innate difference model, biological or psychological differences are credited to inheritance and are, therefore, considered irremediable.[3]

Personal Contexts of Latino Youth

Face-to-face interactions within the microsystem, such as those represented in daily activity settings, like parenting practices in the home and family, and formal and informal spiritual practices, provide the most interpersonally intimate transmission of culture. An understanding and appreciation of the patterning of these interactions among Latino youth is essential to developing culturally responsive interventions.

Parenting Practices in Latino Families

Early development is largely shaped by the parenting practices in the home environment. Even though it is not possible to provide an adequate canvassing of parenting practices among the Latino groups because of the number of Latino subgroups (Mexican, Cuban, Puerto Rican, and so on) and intranational variations (such as the Tarahumara Indians of Chihuahua, the mestizos of Jalisco, and the Spanish elite of Merida in Mexico) and because parenting practices are always undergoing change, this section of the chapter attempts to draw attention to how parenting practices affect development and must be taken into account when designing psychological interventions.

Dependence as Culturally Relative

In an address to the American Psychological Association, developmental psychologist Patricia M. Greenfield began with a story. She described a West Los Angeles elementary school's experience with Latino youth in a federally funded breakfast program.[4] The teachers at the school expressed anger and concern that the mothers of the Latino students brought their younger children to partake of the breakfast, a benefit for which only the enrolled student was entitled according to the federal program. Furthermore, the teachers believed that the Latino mothers prevented the independent development of their school-age children by physically helping them eat.

Greenfield highlighted the need to understand the Latino mothers' values of sharing and caregiving upon which their behavior was based rather to view their behavior as exploiting the federally funded program and inappropriately enabling dependent behavior. The teachers' view of the Latino mothers' behavior toward their school-age children was based on the teachers' own values of individualism and autonomy. As long as the teachers could not appreciate the views and values of Latino families, they were unable to resolve the apparent (to the teachers) problematic behavior of the mothers.

Socialization and Language

In a study of parental reports of child-rearing practices in non-Latino white families, African American families, and Mexican American families, investigators found that poor Mexican American parents were less authoritarian, less achievement-oriented, more protective, and less emphatic about individual responsibility than poor African American or non-Latino white parents.[5] However, some differences that initially appear to be ethnic in nature are the result of other factors, such as education. For example, Robert A. LeVine and his colleagues found that Mexican mothers with more formal education were more verbally responsive to their babies at five, ten, and fifteen months but held their babies less at fifteen months of age.[6] They also found that maternal education was related to a mother's skill in using language that is not connected to a social or pragmatic situation (which they called *decontextualized language*).[7] Such language skill predicts academic performance in other settings.[8] They further noted that the higher the mother's educational level, the more likely she was to take the baby with her and the less likely she was to leave the baby alone or in the care of an older sibling.[9] LeVine and his colleagues present an evolutionary perspective that these changing patterns represent a change in survival strategies that are a response to improving conditions in their societies; for example, better medical facilities, clean water, and so on allow mothers to take their babies with them without fear of their getting sick.

Parental Expectations and Child-Rearing Values

Luis H. Zayas and Fabiana Solari summarize the research on early childhood socialization in Hispanic families.[10] They suggest that Hispanic parents differ from parents of other ethnic groups in child-rearing values and practices when it comes to the interpersonal behavior they expect from their children at home and at school.

Among the examples cited from various studies they reviewed are these: Puerto Rican mothers preferred a quiet child who seeks closeness, whereas Anglo-American mothers preferred an active child; Puerto Rican mothers described their toddlers' behaviors in terms of "relatedness, respectfulness, and affection" whereas Anglo-American mothers described their toddlers' behaviors in terms of "autonomy, personal development, and self-control"; Mexican parents considered noncognitive social skills to be as important as or more important than cognitive skills, whereas Anglo-American parents considered cognitive skills to be more important; Chicano, Puerto Rican, and Dominican mothers used more modeling, visual cues, and directives in teaching their children, whereas Anglo-American mothers used more verbal inquiry and praise; and finally, Puerto Rican mothers and Mexican parents preferred that their children be obedient, follow rules, and conform at school, whereas Anglo-American teachers and parents preferred children to be independent, verbally expressive, and self-directed.

Acculturation and Parenting Practices

Some parenting practices change through acculturation, that is, the adoption of customs, beliefs, and values of the dominant society. Delgado-Gaitan showed that *collectivism* (valuing the welfare of the family or community) is more characteristic of first- or immigrant-generation Mexican Americans than of the second generation.[11] Although the first generation emphasized this value, socialization practices shifted toward an individualistic orientation, especially in the areas of critical thinking. Nonetheless, both generations maintained a strong orientation toward respect and family ties. In a study of healthy eating habits in Mexican American children, the most acculturated mothers used the most forceful child-rearing techniques (like direct imperatives toward the child, threats, lack of choices, and repetition of commands) and fewer nondirective techniques (like hints and questions).[12]

Attention to such proximal processes as parenting practices needs to take both context (such as country of origin, rural or urban area, socioeconomic status) and time (such as generational status or the course of industrialization of a country) into consideration.

There is no easy prescription for defining a Latino family as one that is nonchanging, hierarchical by age and gender, and fostering respect, obedience, and less independence, and so on. Yet stereotypes abound in the social sciences literature.[13]

Spirituality in Latino Families

A number of authors have focused on the role of spirituality among Latinos.[14] Spirituality traverses wide terrain, from formal religion (often Catholicism), to folk religions like Santería, Espiritismo, and Curanderismo, to popular religiosity, to religious community practices, to a much more pervasive spiritualized cosmology. Folk religions have received much attention from anthropologists and other social scientists, but spirituality has a much broader impact. Spirituality among Latinos varies greatly. Caribbean Latinos are distinct in their spirituality from Central American Latinos and South American Latinos. Among South American Latinos, Peruvians differ considerably from Argentines.

Popular Religion Versus Communitarian Spirituality

Ana María Díaz-Stevens believes that spirituality plays different roles for Latinos in their countries of origin than in the United States. She points out that, unlike the United States, Latin America is largely composed of "smaller, poorer, and less developed societies with Catholic majorities and a closer connection to agricultural economies that are dominated by a small ruling class." She suggests that in the United States, "Latinos find a way to define themselves as an ethnic group; in Latin America, on the other hand, popular religiosity is the vehicle for a town or region to affirm itself."[15] Thus, she distinguishes between *popular religiosity* practiced in the Latin American countries of origin, which she believes draws boundaries that are territorial or class-based, and the Latino popular religiosity practiced in this country, which she refers to as *communitarian spirituality* and which she believes creates and reaffirms social bonds between social classes in a particular community. She believes that popular religiosity in Latin American communities provides a means for affirmation of the community itself, whereas communitarian spirituality provides an avenue for a group to define itself as an ethnic group.

An example of popular religiosity in Latin America is the *fiesta patronal*, which mobilizes a community around the celebration of a particular saint. For instance, in the small village of San Lorenzo in Coahuila, Mexico, *Las Fiestas de San Lorenzo* not only commemorate San Lorenzo (the saint) but also unite the village and reaffirm the community.

From our perspective, spirituality is transmitted through proximal processes within different contexts. We believe that spirituality serves the two functions described by Díaz-Stevens regardless of geographic location, although we also believe that Latino popular religiosity becomes a stronger vehicle for identity formation in the United States than in Latin America.

Religious Socialization

The impact of spirituality on the socialization of Latino children is evident in many activities and practices of Latino youth and their families. Parents may take their children to church, but they model spirituality in many other ways. The mother who takes her children on a pilgrimage to a nearby chapel during Holy Week, the family that prays and makes offerings to a saint that is circulated to all families in a community, the mother who takes her child to an *espiritista* or *curandero*, the father who takes his son to the *morada* (a special chapel where *penitentes* practice) to induct him as a *penitente*—all are transmitting potent messages not only about beliefs but more importantly about practices, interpersonal relationships (such as how to behave toward parents, neighbors, and elders), and gender and ethnic identity.

Spirituality and Formal Religion

Joseph M. Cervantes and Oscar Ramírez have drawn attention to the role of spirituality, as separate from practice of a formal religion, in Mexican American families. The authors proposed that Mexican Americans have a psychospiritual perspective that they call *mestizo spirituality*, which influences how children are raised. According to Cervantes and Ramírez, Mexican American children are oriented to life within the immediate and extended family as "a protective sanctuary," taught to value generational wisdom, and instilled with belief in the interconnectedness of all life and a "theistic cosmology that protects, influences, and engages all of life."[16]

They illustrate through case examples how issues of spirituality need to be taken into account in family therapy.

Apart from the practice of formal religion, issues of spirituality are often ignored in both clinical and developmental psychology. Yet such issues are central to many Latino families—either because the family embraces a spirituality typical of its cultural group or because it is actively denying the spirituality typical of its cultural group. However, as already noted, Latinos vary widely in their spirituality. For example, *La Virgen de Guadalupe* is a potent symbol for Mexican Americans, as we mentioned in Chapter Two. The statue is more than a symbol of Catholicism to them. In many ways, *La Virgen* makes more sense when seen from the Indian perspective. She is clearly Indian in features and complexion. She stands on the moon wearing a blue shawl with stars, and she holds her hands not in the Western European tradition of prayer but according to the Indian custom of placing the hands together before making an important announcement—all of which symbolizes that she is about to make an announcement of cosmic proportion. Any Indian knows what that announcement is. She wears a pregnancy sash and Indians know of the prophecy that a new race was to be born. With the arrival of the Spaniards, the new race was the mestizo race—the offspring of the marriage of Indian and Spanish cultures.[17]

Many Puerto Ricans, Dominicans, and Cubans carry out community and family rituals based in a belief system that includes Afro-Caribbean gods originating from West and Central Africa and syncretized with Catholic saints. Popular or folk religion as well as established church practices differ across Latino cultures. However, in all of the Latin American cultures, belief in spirits of recent or ancient deceased persons is expressed in parallel practices and a popular folk religion in which spirit mediums divine and heal.[18] Children are not explicitly taught to believe in spirits, but they learn about these beliefs by observing parents worshiping at home altars or in family or community séances. Caribbean Latino parents model for their children how to be spiritual but usually do not dictate participation in a particular established religion or folk practice.[19] Fundamentalist Protestant Latino families are often the exception. Children in Puerto Rico are explicitly conceded the freedom to choose their own form of spirituality if it more or less conforms to the mores and values of the family.[20]

Of particular relevance to our discussion of spirituality is the frequency with which God, angels, and saints are invoked. It is almost automatic for most Latinos to call on God in a situation of danger, and it is common for persons of Mexican and Central American descent (especially the less acculturated) to invoke God to protect them against an uncertain future. *Si Dios quiere* (If God wills it) or *Que Dios nos bendiga* (May God bless us) often preface embarking on new journeys and new experiences. There may also be the fear of evil lurking in the background, particularly a fear of the *mal (de) ojo* (the evil eye), most often perpetrated unknowingly by someone admiring or envying something beautiful—whether a material possession or a small child.

There are folk rhymes in which children ask for God's protection when they have a new thing of value, and mothers commonly pin small amulets (*medallas, escapularios,* or *azabaches*) to their babies' undershirts to safeguard them from illness. It makes no difference that these folkways can be traced to combined Native American, Afro-Caribbean, and folk Spanish traditions; they transcend the borders of diverse Latino cultures. When one of our ex-students, a Latina who had become a psychologist on the faculty of a university, gave birth to a daughter, one of us sent her a tiny silver bracelet with a coral stone made by a Pueblo Indian in New Mexico. The coral represents the main element of the *azabache* amulet. It was gracefully accepted by the baby's nonbeliever mother, because the child's Dominican nurse had been urging her to get proper protection for her baby!

The Case of Lucia

The case of Lucia provides another example of the impact of spirituality on the development not only of spiritual beliefs but also of social relations, moral beliefs, and gender and ethnic identity in a Latina girl.

> Lucia, a fourteen-year-old Mexican American girl, is brought to therapy by her aunt, who has custody of her. A year earlier, her parents died in a car accident on their way to work the fields in California and Oregon. Recently, Lucia has become increasingly depressed and withdrawn and has received failing grades in all but two subjects on her report card. Lucia's aunt is very Americanized, and she has stopped many cultural practices that Lucia enjoyed when she lived with her parents.

Lucia is still grieving the death of her parents. As she describes her grief, Lucia tells the clinician how she missed not celebrating Christmas in the way her family did. She missed preparing the tamales with "all the women" on Christmas Eve, going to midnight mass where she used to see her friends and they would all roll their eyes at one another to commiserate about having to be there, and eating the tamales with *champurado* (a thick chocolate-flavored drink made with cornmeal) in a festive celebration at her grandparents' house. During the *tamalada* (the making of the tamales), she had learned much about relationships with adults and peers, about gender-related behaviors, about skills she would need when she gets married. At one point, she laments that she even misses going with her mother to light votive candles for some special petition. During these times, she had learned about what was going on in the immediate and extended family and also enjoyed the special camaraderie with her mother. With eyes welling with tears, she says, "I hope I can be the way she wanted me to be, but I don't know if I had time to learn all the right things," while making the sign of the cross. She then tells the clinician that at night she prays to her mother's patron saint and, on Sundays when her aunt takes her to church, asks her aunt to go with her to light a votive candle in memory of her mother. "It's funny," she says, as she fingers the scapular of *El Santo Niño de Praga* that her father gave her, "but my aunt thinks I'm too old-fashioned. I just don't fit in her family."

Gender, Racial, and Ethnic Identity

Proximal processes shape gender, racial, and ethnic identity. Most clinicians are well aware that although gender identity occurs at a young age, racial and ethnic identity not only require more time but also can develop with considerable turmoil. The case of Gabby, the teenager we described in Chapter One, illustrates how difficult ethnic identity struggles can be. Gabby's identification with the goth and darkwave cultures of middle-class, disenfranchised non-Latino youth is in part a rebellion against her father, who is trying to prevent her from losing her heritage as he did, when he was her age.

A review of the empirical literature demonstrates that ethnic awareness and ethnic self-identification develop considerably later than gender and race awareness and self-identification.[21] Martha E. Bernal, George Knight, and their colleagues have summarized studies in these areas.[22] Gender awareness is acquired by most children (70 percent of them) approximately between the ages of two and just over three, race awareness between ages four and five, and ethnicity awareness between five and ten. Gender self-identification is acquired by most children (70 percent of them) approximately between just over age two and age four, race self-identification between ages three and seven, and ethnic self-identification between ages seven and ten. However, racial and ethnic constancies, which refer to the knowledge that one's own racial and ethnic characteristics are permanent and cannot change over time or context, occur after mastery of gender constancy. Whereas gender constancy is achieved by the majority of children (70 percent of them) approximately between the ages of four and a half and seven, race constancy is achieved between ages eight and eleven, and ethnic constancy between eight and ten.

In discussing these research findings, these investigators underscore the limitations of the cognitive developmental framework, particularly its failure to explain the delay of racial and ethnic identity formation in children who possess the necessary mental structure otherwise to understand physical constancies. They offer an information-processing perspective to account for the sequencing of the acquisition of gender, racial, and ethnic identity. We suggest that a contextual model can also account for the sequencing and that such sequencing in our U.S. society is the result of an interaction among several factors: biopsychological processes (the information processing hypothesized by Bernal and her colleagues, for example); proximal processes (socialization by parents and significant caregivers); context (the salience of racial and ethnic issues in a community); and time (the 1990s versus the 1950s).

Although physical attributes assist in defining male from female, and skin color and facial features are used to distinguish among the so-called races, ethnic identity is more difficult to characterize. A further complication to racial and ethnic identity is that an increasing number of youth are of mixed racial and ethnic backgrounds. For these children, it is difficult to establish what the ethnic identity ideally should be, as is the case with Gabby. In Mexican and other Central American families, children are sometimes viewed differently depending on how dark their complexion is or how Indian their features are; those tending more toward the Indian are usually not viewed as positively. Among Caribbean Latinos, families make references to such characteristics as *pelo malo* (bad hair, referring to African kinky hair) to denote the presence of African characteristics. As the *pelo malo* example illustrates, these characteristics are not viewed favorably either. Thus, for a child with Indian or African features, growing up in a Latino family may be a different experience from that of fairer-skinned, Caucasian-featured siblings. Because these issues are more likely acted upon than spoken about in a family, the contextual clinician must be astute in observing the nonverbal and indirect verbal communications in the family. Gender identity is usually influenced primarily by biopsychological aspects (genitalia and other physical attributes) within the individual because proximal processes, although still important, usually do not shape gender identity as much as biopsychological characteristics do. (Some exceptions may be the development of homosexuality and transvestism.) However, racial identity and ethnic identity usually require much greater influence than gender identity of aspects other than biopsychological ones, namely, proximal processes (parent-child and family relationships, for example), context (country of residence or the neighborhood in which the child lives), and time (growing up in East Los Angeles in the 1970s when the Chicano movement was very active, for example). The following case illustrates the importance of proximal processes, context, and time in the emerging ethnic identity of a preadolescent.

> Jaime is an eleven-year-old Cuban boy who came to the United States with his mother and sister about two years ago. He proudly talks about his numerous "girlfriends." His mother finds amusement in his male precociousness, smiling at the clinician as Jaime describes his "conquests." She does nothing to deflate his valuation of his sexuality and, in fact, encourages it. "Even young women in their late teens and early twenties find him attractive," she says in Spanish. Jaime inflates his chest and raises his head high. While she complains that Jaime is getting too raucous at school and is getting into too many fights both at school and in the neighborhood, she smiles at him as she makes eye contact, and says to the clinician: *"¡Es puro varón!"* ("He is all boy!") Jaime's enhanced, almost caricatured masculinity is fueled by his mother's interactions with him. However, Jaime speaks to his mother, who speaks almost no English, and to the clinician solely in English. In his broken, heavily accented English, he tells the clinician: "Oh man, I forget all my Spanish!" In English, he complains about the clothes his mother buys him and expresses his strong preference for baggy clothes and expensive brand-name tennis

shoes. As he speaks, he uses gestures typical of rap artists. His mother exclaims: *"¿Que es esto? ¿Te crees Negro o cholo?"* ("What is this? You think you are black or a Latino street youth?") At eleven, Jaime does not want to be either a Cuban or a Spanish speaker: "Oh man, she need to chill out. It's not Cuba!"

Are racial and ethnic identity important to the development of emotional and behavioral problems as well as to interventions to address these problems? We believe that racial and ethnic identity are important areas of focus both in assessing problems and in finding effective interventions for them. Another well-known researcher on racial and ethnic identity, Jean S. Phinney, stresses the need to have adolescents explore their culture in order to help them understand its strengths and accept not only their culture but themselves.[23] She believes that adolescents who achieve a positive ethnic identity can better deal with negative stereotypes and prejudice and not internalize negative self-perceptions, and that a positive ethnic identity contributes to better psychological adjustment.

Language and Its Influence on Development

Language affects children in two general ways: through its content (what it means) and through its process (how it is used).

Language Content

An example of the influence of language content on development is provided by Sabine Ulibarri, a noted southwestern author.[24] During a lecture at one of our seminars on providing mental health services to culturally diverse youths and their families, Ulibarri made the point that North Americans "run around with women" while Latinos "walk with them" (*andan con ellas*). The Latino idea of walking with women probably dates back to the time when young women walked around the plaza, chaperoned by a family member, to be viewed by the marriageable young men, who also walked around the plaza. If Latino male adolescents are socialized to "walk" with their girlfriends and North American males to "run" with them, their experience of boy-girl relationships is apt to be quite different. In another example, a Cuban colleague once noted during a lecture on Latino families that there is no Spanish term for *toilet training* and speculated on the overvaluation of toilet training and its hypothesized role in numerous developmental processes in North American society.[25]

Do certain languages lend themselves to metaphor and the potent and evocative use of symbolism? We believe so. Precise languages like English and German that have words for most things may be well suited to applying the scientific method, to developing operational and parsimonious definitions. They may have been well suited to take countries into the industrial age. However, this precision can detract from the use of metaphor. Precise meaning may come at the expense of evocative meaning that draws from the affective experience of both the speaker and the listener. In contrast to English, Spanish appears less precise yet more powerful with regard to the emotions its words can elicit. If English is the language of the scientist, Spanish is the language of the poet. The English-speaking clinician conducting therapy with a bilingual Latino whose preferred language is Spanish may be like the scientist trying to reason with the poet. The language of the poet is likely to leave the scientist befuddled, if not frustrated.

How language is used is equally important. As Spanish-speaking Latinos learn English, we, as contextual clinicians, cannot underestimate the temporal aspects of change in language use and preference. As another colleague, Artemio Brambila, often points out, the language a person spoke as a child and the language that is used when that person comes for therapy is a factor often ignored by many therapists.[26] In the case of a teenager or adult who may now be primarily English-speaking but whose first language was Spanish, the cognitive and affective experience associated with an event he or she had as a child will likely be considerably attenuated if it is recalled in English. The memory of an experience in the person's native language is rich and evocative, but the same memory in the language acquired after the experience can be insipid.

Another aspect of how language is used is illustrated in studies of mother-child interactions. Studies of these interactions often code the types of statements that the mother makes to her child into discrete categories. In one study, verbal behavior of the mothers was divided into *syntactic directives* (using hints, asking questions, requesting permission, giving imperatives, and so on), *semantic directives* (minimizing the task, justifying an activity, bargaining, expressing affection, giving praise, and so on), and *semantic aggravators* (threatening punishment, not allowing choices of activities, emphatically repeating statements, and so on).[27] Communication by the parent to the child emphasizing any of these three categories may lead to a child feeling valued and competent, disparaged and ineffective, or misunderstood and exploited; it may leave the child feeling proud and happy, or sad and angry.

Socialization and Language

There is ample evidence that Latino children have a rich verbal folklore consisting of poems, sayings, chants, riddles, rhymes, and jingles invoked by them or by adults in particular situations.[28] Among Puerto Rican children, for example, these forms of communication regulate relationships between youths in neighborhood games and assist young children in acquiring cognitive skills, such as reciting the alphabet or identifying body parts. Metaphor is commonly used in the Spanish language to regulate affective, instrumental, and moral behavior. *Dichos* (proverbs), a common use of metaphor, are frequently interposed in adult-child discourse and repeated in peer interactions. When a Latino youngster was eager to go home from the hospital following his understanding that he had made many positive behavior changes, his mother cautioned, *"No puedes tapar el cielo con la mano"* ("You cannot cover the sky with your hand"). In other words: don't try to do too much and overreach, everything will happen in due time.

In a study of mainland Puerto Rican children, it was found that family members, both nuclear and extended, had taught more of the stories and riddles than had peers or schoolteachers.[29] This may be the result of dangerous neighborhoods and confinement of young children to the home, which is common in urban environments. In contrast, in rural settings in Latin American countries of origin, less formal transmission of cultural themes for behavior and belief traditionally comes from adults. The themes noted for mainland Puerto Rican verbal folklore were motherly love and affection, great affection for babies, gender role distinctions, lovers and romance, tricks, retorts and taunts, spirituality, threatening figures meant to control children's behavior (*el cuco* in Puerto Rico and *la llorona* in Mexico and the U.S. Southwest border areas), magical forces, and closeness to nature through encounters with animals or idyllic natural settings. The last is an integral part of the rural experience of Puerto Rican and most Latin American cultures.

The Cultural Construction of the Self in the United States

The conceptualization of the individual—or the self—in the United States is culturally rooted, as it is across the world. Yet we often assume that the U.S. conceptualization of the self is the only viable one. We have based much of our presumably universal psychology about the individual on this conceptualization. Various authors have presented cogent arguments about the need to consider psychologies that are not so focused on the individual.[30] They have questioned the underlying beliefs emphasized by the dominant U.S. society, which assert firm boundaries between self and other; personal or internal locus of control by which the self acts upon the world and others to meet its needs; and a separate, encapsulated self. Hope Landrine points out that, in the U.S. conceptualization of the self, "the self is presumed to be a free agent" with inalienable rights, such as "the right to privacy, autonomy, and to be protected from intrusions from others." She further notes that, within this conceptualization of the self, failure to seek control is seen to be passive, helpless, unassertive, submissive, and indicative of low self-esteem, feelings of inadequacy, and even depression.[31] Underscoring that psychology is not immune from the insidious effects of political and cultural values, Edward E. Sampson described how the past two presidential addresses to the American Psychological Association, given several years before the publication of his article, argued strongly "in support of the fundamental and beneficial quality of the American character, its individualism."[32]

Relevance to Latino Youth

Both Sampson and Landrine propose a different conceptualization of the self that is more compatible with that of many American ethnic minorities, including Latinos. This alternative conceptualization assumes much more fluid self-other boundaries, views control as extending beyond the self into the environment, considers the self to be defined by its relationships and contexts, and does *not* view the self as a separate, bounded, masterful entity.

The Cultural Construction of the Self in Latin America

The alternative conceptualization of the self offered by Sampson and Landrine more aptly describes the Latino, as well as the Latin American, conceptualization of the self. We have emphasized that Latinos vary widely both in the United States and in their countries of origin. The mestizo *campesino* from the deserts of northern Mexico seems to share little with the mulatto fisherman from the coast of Colombia or the Spanish-Italian *finca* owner from Argentina. The Mexican *maquiladora* worker, the *ladino* shop owner from Guatemala, and the *descamisados* from Argentina on the surface seem, both literally and figuratively, worlds apart. Yet Latinos may have more in common in the way they conceptualize the self. In part, this may be related to their socioeconomic and political history, which we discussed in Chapter One. Latin American countries retain a close historical tie to rural and agricultural economies, which value a communitarian ideology predicated on the interdependence of individuals in the community. In part, the Latino view of the self may also have been formed with the influence of Native American ideologies and cosmologies in Central and South American countries and the influence of African ideologies and cosmologies in Caribbean Latin American countries. Native American and African cultures view the self as inextricably embedded in larger contexts, and consequently control is external to the self. The self must maintain a certain harmony or balance with nature or the physical and social contexts in which a person lives.

A Sociohistorical Perspective

A contextual approach to intervention requires that we take into consideration the impact of historical events and conditions (parents having escaped from a war-torn country or having lived in villages that had strong communitarian values, or the child experiencing discrimination and abject poverty, for example) on the child and his or her immediate context (at home, in the neighborhood, or at school). Philip Cushman cogently argues for a historically situated psychology. He posits that the self in the United States has been conceptualized as a "bounded, masterful self; an unchangeable, transhistorical self."[33] Other authors describe prevalent European American notions of self-contained individualism and the referential self[34] in ways that closely parallel Cushman's formulation. Cushman notes that, in the face of changing economies and politics in the post–World War II era, the current version of the bounded masterful self is the empty self: "By this I mean that our terrain has shaped a self that experiences a significant absence of community, tradition, and shared meaning. It experiences these social absences and their consequences 'interiorly' as a lack of personal conviction and worth, and it embodies the absences as a chronic, undifferentiated emotional hunger. The post–World War II self thus yearns to acquire and consume as an unconscious way of compensating for what has been lost: It is empty."[35]

What we are witnessing in today's North American youth may be the consequence of generations of purging America's multicultural population of its diverse ethnicities and their cultures: the homogenization of America that Schwarz has described.[36] As clinicians, we are frequently confronted with youths seeking meaning and connection with others. They ironically identify with idealized heroes and heroines in films such as *The Raven* and *Pulp Fiction* who symbolize Cushman's empty self and are desperately fighting intense feelings of alienation and fragmentation.

A social constructionist view—one that assumes that where we are situated in time and those with whom we interact in our immediate and remote cultural practices define who we are at a given moment—is compatible with our contextual framework for selecting and developing psychological interventions. We can define and experience ourselves only at a given moment in time. The youths we treat today are very different from the youths of their parents' generation. Latino parents face two significant problems. Like their dominant-culture counterparts, they must attempt to understand the ethos of today's youth. Unlike their dominant-culture counterparts, they must make sense of their children's cultural conflicts that arise through ethnic interrelationships. But Latino youth also confront two significant problems. They must deal with their parents' concepts of appropriate child rearing, which are rooted in different experiences, and they must also deal with cultural conflicts between themselves and dominant-culture youth. Gabby, our earlier example, struggles to find "her place" among the dominant-culture youth with whom she associates. But she must also deal with her father's efforts to bring her up like a "traditional Mexican teenager" who, ironically, no longer exists in Mexican society, where the current adolescent generation is considerably different from the preceding generation known to her father. Our efforts to understand a young Latino or Latina with problems may also be made more difficult by our formal systems of diagnosing emotional and behavioral problems in youth.

Limitations of Noncontextual Models of Psychopathology

North American society has many mental health conventions and practices that attempt to dictate how we go about our task of diagnosing and treating so-called mental disorders. Most clinicians in our mental health service community have long espoused an individual-centered diagnostic system—the *Diagnostic and Statistical Manual of Mental Disorders,* currently in its fourth version (DSM-IV)—that places the etiology of a mental disorder within the individual.[37] In fact, the DSM-IV is the standard that is required by Medicaid, Medicare, most insurance companies, and most managed care organizations. The DSM-IV is very consistent with our Western European and North American worldviews, where the individual-centered approach to diagnosis predominates in clinical and research practice. Yet such an approach, particularly when used to assess children and adolescents with behavioral and emotional problems, continues to be fraught with difficulties. How does one understand a child or adolescent apart from his proximal processes (interactions with his parents, peers, teachers, and so on) and contexts (family, neighborhood, and school)?

Research on how mental health problems in Latinos are evaluated by clinicians shows that culture influences psychiatric diagnosis in the assessment of symptoms, in the configuration of symptoms into disorders, and in the interpersonal interaction of the client and the diagnostician.[38] Lloyd H. Rogler has recommended that the pretesting phase in culturally responsive research be expanded to include spending time with the group to be studied, preferably using traditional methods of descriptive anthropology that involve participant observation and interviews with key informants who are knowledgeable about specific aspects of their culture.[39] Two decades ago, A. J. Marsella, another well-known cross-cultural researcher, advocated conducting empirical studies of the conceptualization of mental health and disorders in different cultures.[40] He suggested developing research matrices for investigating problems, causes, and treatment interactions in different cultures. In essence, Rogler and Marsella were advocating research approaches that are more contextual. Rogler's recommendation for participant observation and interviews with informants encourages clinicians to learn about important proximal face-to-face interactions that shape the lives of the subjects under study. It is also a recommendation to researchers to craft their investigation by allowing themselves to learn about a group under study by interacting with its members face to face.

Language differences also play an important role in diagnosing.[41] According to studies on differences in diagnosis depending on the language in which diagnostic interviews are conducted and the client's degree of fluency in it, the language used during the evaluation affects diagnostic outcomes.[42] One investigator found that diagnosticians were more likely to infer that the client has more severe mental illness when a primarily Spanish-speaking client reports his or her symptoms in English.[43]

Even if certain types of psychiatric disorders are shown to have a biochemical basis, an individual experiencing a mental disorder must still interpret the abnormal experience, translate the experience into behavior, and respond to the social reaction to that behavior.[44] An accurate assessment of a problem requires a contextual approach in which the focus of evaluation is not just the individual but rather the individual-in-activity-in-a-context (as in Vygotsky's model); the person-participating-in-a-cultural practice (as in Cole's conceptualization); or the interaction among proximal processes, the person, context, and time (as in Bronfenbrenner's model).

Understanding a Youth's Problems from a Contextual Framework

To the degree that a contextual perspective addresses the interplay between the biopsychological individual and the varied contexts in which he or she lives, the very term *psychopathology* becomes a misnomer. Psychopathology implies a focus on problems intrinsic to the individual and devoid of contextual contributions to or interrelationships with the problems. As was discussed in Chapter Two, the focus of a contextual model is on the interplay between the developing individual and varied activities in varied contexts at varied times. Assessment and intervention within the microsystem requires attention to the specific biopsychological characteristics of Latino youth that speak both to their strengths and problems, to the nature and quality of the proximal processes they have and are experiencing, to the specific contexts in which they navigate, and to the influence of sociohistorical events as they bear on both proximal processes and the immediate environment.

To illustrate, getting involved in a gang may be seen simply as a manifestation of a conduct disorder or, in part, as a way for certain Latino adolescents to separate from their families of origin and resolve certain identity crises and family conflicts.[45] James Diego Vigil described the common identity crisis in Chicano adolescent gang members.[46] Because many of these adolescents come from disorganized and troubled families that cannot meet the children's psychosocial needs, and because they have limited involvement with community resources and limited access to positive role models, the older gang members, or *veteranos,* serve as role models for them. According to Vigil, these youths adopt and internalize the behaviors, values, and attitudes of the *veteranos.* At the same time, they consolidate their identification with the aggressor at home and continue to have an increasingly conflictual relationship with their mothers. Some clinicians suggest that "gang members are counterparts who validate and legitimatize each other's experientially and culturally determined concepts of masculinity" and that "affiliation with the gang provides these youths with a reference group, which allows them to integrate the negative aspects of themselves into a newly constructed self-identity."[47]

We should caution about assuming a deficiency or deficit model under the guise of contextualism. The deficiency or deficit model compares ethnic minority children with middle-class children of the dominant culture and their biological, psychological, or intellectual differences are attributed to cultural deprivation caused by poverty, poorly educated parents, or other environmental conditions at odds with the ideal conditions associated with child development in the dominant cultural group.[48] The reason we do not consider these contextual models is that the assessment of the "minority" group is made from the views and values of the "majority." The definition of competencies as outcomes of development must be changed from that which the dominant society's standards (established in studies of predominantly white middle-class youth) deem optimal to that which assist minority youth to cope constructively with the sociocultural contexts in which they participate.

Changes in Individual-Based Diagnosis Conducive to Contextual Approaches

The recognition of the need to incorporate a contextual framework has been growing in clinical practice. We believe that this reflects a growing awareness that individual-based diagnosis is insufficient both in obtaining an adequate assessment of problems individuals have and in developing effective interventions that generalize across the different contexts in which individuals live. We will focus on two examples. About twenty years ago, Jane Mercer introduced the System of Multicultural Pluralistic Assessment (SOMPA) to take into account broader contextual aspects—like adaptive functioning, which describes a variety of daily skills—in the assessment of intelligence of minority youth.[49] Her effort was the result of studies showing that certain ethnic minority groups were being assessed as lower-functioning than they might actually be. Considering information from contexts other than the testing situation alone gave a more representative view of a minority child's actual skills, abilities, and competencies. Similarly, it has become the standard of practice to use both an intelligence test and a measure of adaptive functioning to assess adequately mental retardation. The notion is that an individual not only must have an IQ in the mentally retarded range but also show a level of adaptive functioning across various domains (such as communication, daily living skills, motor skills, and socialization) that is commensurate with the IQ score. If the level of adaptive behavior is too high, the individual cannot be said to be mentally retarded.

The second example of the growing awareness of the limitations of individual-based diagnosis and the need to incorporate contextual aspects of the problem comes from a more recent change in how we view psychiatric diagnosis and the need for service. Recently, it has been recognized that diagnosis alone (which is a product of symptom configuration and symptom severity and "resides" within the individual) is not sufficient to determine the need for services. Diagnosis along with level of impairment justify need for service. In the third revision of the DSM, a multiaxial approach was used.[50] Although the first three axes focused on individual-based disorders or conditions, Axis IV described psychosocial stressors and their severity, and Axis V was a global assessment of functioning that reflected the current need for treatment or care. Two very large multisite National Institute of Mental Health (NIMH) studies, one begun in the 1980s and the other in the 1990s, use the concept of diagnosis plus impairment. The first study, the NIMH Methods for the Epidemiology of Child and Adolescent Mental Disorders (MECA) study, established the methodology to be used in the subsequent and larger NIMH Study of the Mental Health Service Use, Need, Outcomes, and Costs in Children and Adolescent Populations (UNOCCAP) currently in progress. These two studies underscore the increasing realization among researchers of the need to incorporate context into assessments of behavioral and emotional problems.

On the surface, the recognition that it is important to determine both diagnosis and level of impairment seems like a continuation of the individual-centered perspective that we have previously critiqued. However, the implications of attending to level of impairment and stressors are noteworthy. Attention to level of impairment and stressors presents a potential check on the applicability of a diagnostic construct to persons from diverse cultures because it requires the clinician to consider a person's actual functioning in the contexts or activity settings in which he or she participates. A Latino youth may appear to have an attention-deficit hyperactivity disorder (ADHD) as assessed by a clinician using standardized normed questionnaires, observations by clinician, and computer-based, standardized, and normed vigilance tests, as was the case in a particular study of Puerto Rican children. In this study, the investigator found that a very high number of Puerto Rican children qualified for a diagnosis of attention-deficit hyperactivity disorder (50 percent of the sample), which is far greater than the prevalence of the disorder (3 percent to 5 percent of school-age children) in the U.S. mainland.[51]

However, if the clinician asked the child's parents or teachers from the same community or culture about their assessment of how impaired that child's functioning in day-to-day activities was, the parents and teachers might say there was no or minimal impairment across activity settings at home and at school. Thus, that child would not be diagnosed as having ADHD. Inclusion of level of impairment to determine both diagnosis and need for service requires evaluation in a more contextual manner. Nonetheless, the approach of DSM-based diagnosis plus impairment is not truly contextual because it uses context as an "add on" to an approach that remains theoretically noncontextual and individual-centered, as we discussed in Chapter Two.

Conclusion

In this chapter we have explored aspects of culture, development, and behavioral and emotional problems within microsystemic contexts—particularly the family and school. We have selectively reviewed topics that we consider central to culturally responsive interventions and have critically discussed current diagnostic practice. Although much current practice in mental health has focused on this level of context, there is increasing dissatisfaction with the delivery of mental health services for youth within this narrow scope. Chapter Four will illustrate the application of contextually based assessment and treatment of Latino youth within microsystemic contexts.

Notes

1. U. Bronfenbrenner, "Developmental Ecology Through Space and Time: A Future Perspective," in *Examining Lives in Context: Perspectives on the Ecology of Human Development,* ed. P. Moen, G. H. Elder Jr., and K. Lüscher (Washington, D.C.: American Psychological Association, 1995).
2. Bronfenbrenner, "Developmental Ecology."
3. C. Garcia Coll and others, "An Integrative Model for the Study of Developmental Competencies in Minority Children," *Child Development, 67* (1996): 1891–1914.
4. P. M. Greenfield, "Conflicting Values in Hispanic Immigrant Families and the Schools," address to the 103rd Annual Convention of the American Psychological Association, New York, 1995.

5. M. E. Durrett, S. O'Bryant, and J. W. Pennebaker, "Childrearing Report of White, Black, and Mexican-American Families," *Developmental Psychology, 2* (1975): 871.

6. R. A. LeVine, S. E. LeVine, A. Richman, F. M. Tapia Uribe, C. S. Correa, and P. M. Miller, "Women's Schooling and Child Care in Demographic Transition: A Mexican Case Study," *Population and Development Review, 17* (1991): 459–496.

7. F. M. Tapia Uribe, R. A. LeVine, and S. E. LeVine, "Maternal Education and Maternal Behaviour in Mexico: Implications for the Changing Characteristics of Mexican Immigrants to the United States," *International Journal of Behavioral Development, 16*(3) (1993): 395–408.

8. C. E. Snow, "The Development of Definitional Skill," *Journal of Child Language, 17* (1990): 697–710.

9. Tapia Uribe, LeVine, and LeVine, "Maternal Education."

10. L. H. Zayas and F. Solari, "Early Childhood Socialization in Hispanic Families: Context, Culture and Practice Implications," *Professional Psychology: Research and Practice, 25*(3) (1994): 200–206.

11. C. Delgado-Gaitan, "Parenting in Two Generations of Mexican American Families," *International Journal of Behavioural Development, 16*(3) (1993): 409–427.

12. J. H. Cousins, T. G. Power, and N. Olvera-Ezzel, "Mexican-American Mothers' Socialization Strategies: Effects of Education, Acculturation, and Health Locus of Control," *Journal of Experimental Child Psychology, 55* (1993): 258–276.

13. S. J. Andrade, "Social Science Stereotypes of the Mexican American Woman: Policy Implications for Research," *Hispanic Journal of Behavioral Sciences, 4* (1982): 223–244.

14. V. De La Cancela and I. Z. Martinez, "An Analysis of Culturalism in Latino Mental Health: Folk Medicine as a Case in Point," *Hispanic Journal of Behavioral Sciences, 5*(3) (1983): 251–274; A. Padilla and N. Salgado de Snyder, "Psychology in Pre-Columbian Mexico," *Hispanic Journal of Behavioral Sciences, 10*(1) (1988): 55–66; D. Landy, *Tropical Childhood* (Chapel Hill: University of North Carolina Press, 1959); M. Ramirez, *Psychology of the Americas* (New York: Pergamon Press, 1983); J. M. Cervantes and O. Ramírez, "Spirituality and Family Dynamics in Psychotherapy with Latino Children," in *Working with Culture: Psychotherapeutic Interventions with Ethnic Minority Children and Adolescents,* ed. L. A. Vargas and J. D. Koss-Chioino (San Francisco: Jossey-Bass, 1992).

15. A. M. Díaz-Stevens, *Latino Popular Religiosity and Communitarian Spirituality,* Program for the Analysis of Religion Among Latinos (PARAL) Occasional Paper no. 4 (Sept. 1996): 1, 2.

16. J. M. Cervantes and O. Ramírez, "Spirituality and Family Dynamics in Psychotherapy with Latino Children," *Working with Culture: Psychotherapeutic Interventions with Ethnic Minority Children and Adolescents,* ed. L. A. Vargas and J. D. Koss-Chioino (San Francisco: Jossey-Bass, 1992), 106.

17. Roberto Gomez, personal communication.

18. J. D. Koss-Chioino, "Traditional and Folk Approaches Among Ethnic Minorities," in *Psychological Intervention and Treatment of Ethnic Minorities,* ed. J. F. Aponte, R. R. Rivers, and J. Wohl (Needham Heights, Mass.: Allyn & Bacon, 1995).

19. J. D. Koss, "Spirits as Socializing Agents: A Case Study of a Puerto Rican Girl Reared in a Matricentric Family," in *Case Studies in Spirit Possession,* ed. V. Garrison and V. Crapanzano (New York: Wiley, 1977).

20. Landy, *Tropical Childhood.*

21. *Ethnic Identity: Formation and Transmission Among Hispanics and Other Minorities,* ed. M. E. Bernal and G. P. Knight (New York: State University of New York Press, 1993); K. A. Ocampo, M. Bernal, and G. P. Knight, "Gender, Race, and Ethnicity: The Sequencing of Social Constancies," in *Ethnic Identity: Formation and Transmission Among Hispanics and Other Minorities,* ed. M. E. Bernal and G. P. Knight (New York: State University of New York Press, 1993).

22. Bernal and Knight, *Ethnic Identity.*

23. J. S. Phinney, "A Three-Stage Model of Ethnic Identity Development in Adolescence," in *Ethnic Identity: Formation and Transmission Among Hispanics and Other Minorities,* ed. M. E. Bernal and G. P. Knight (New York: State University of New York Press, 1993).

24. S. Ulibarri, "Differences and Similarities Between Spanish/Mexican and Anglo Cultures," guest lecture presented at the Multicultural Seminar, Division of Child and Adolescent Psychiatry, University of New Mexico Children's Psychiatric Hospital, Albuquerque, N.M. (Apr. 2, 1985).

25. José M. Cañive, personal communication.

26. Artemio De Dios Brambila, personal communication.

27. Cousins, Power, and Olvera-Ezzel, "Mexican-American Mothers."

28. K. Hill, "The Verbal Folklore of Puerto Rican Children: Implications for Promoting School Achievement," in *Puerto Rican Children in the Mainland: Interdisciplinary Perspectives,* ed. A. N. Ambert and M. D. Alvarez (New York: Garland Press, 1992).

29. Hill, "The Verbal Folklore."

30. E. E. Sampson, "The Debate on Individualism: Indigenous Psychologies of the Individual and Their Role in Personal and Societal Functioning," *American Psychologist, 43* (1988): 15–22; H. Landrine,

"Clinical Implications of Cultural Differences: The Referential Versus Indexical Self," *Clinical Psychology Review, 12* (1992): 401–414.

31. Landrine, "Clinical Implications."
32. Sampson, "The Debate on Individualism."
33. P. Cushman, "Why the Self Is Empty: Toward a Historically Situated Psychology," *American Psychologist, 45*(5) (1990): 599–611.
34. Sampson, "The Debate on Individualism."
35. Cushman, "Why the Self Is Empty," p. 600.
36. B. Schwarz, "The Diversity Myth: America's Leading Export," *Atlantic Monthly* (May 1995): 57–67.
37. American Psychiatric Association, *Diagnostic and Statistical Manual of Mental Disorders*, 4th ed. (Washington, D.C.: American Psychiatric Association, 1994).
38. L. H. Rogler, "Research on Mental Health Services for Hispanics: Targets of Convergence," *Cultural Diversity and Mental Health, 2*(3) (1996): 145–556.
39. L. H. Rogler, "The Meaning of Culturally Sensitive Research in Mental Health," *American Journal of Psychiatry, 146* (1989): 296–303.
40. A. J. Marsella, "Cross-Cultural Studies of Mental Health," in *Perspectives on Cross-Cultural Psychology*, ed. A. J. Marsella, R. G. Tharp, and T. J. Ciborowski (New York: Academic Press, 1979).
41. A. J. Marsella, "Depressive Experience and Disorder Across Cultures," in *Handbook of Cross-Cultural Psychology*, vol. 1, *Psychopathology*, ed. H. C. Triandis and J. G. Draguns (Needham Heights, Mass.: Allyn & Bacon, 1980).
42. Rogler, "Research on Mental Health Services."
43. L. R. Marcos, L. Urcuyo, M. Kesselman, and M. Alpert, "The Language Barrier in Evaluating Spanish-American Patients," *Archives of General Psychiatry, 29* (1973): 655–659.
44. A. J. Marsella, N. Sartorius, A. Jablensky, and F. R. Fenton, "Cross-Cultural Studies of Depressive Disorders: An Overview," in *Culture and Depression*, ed. A. Kleinman and B. Good (Berkeley: University of California Press, 1985).
45. J. Belitz and D. M. Valdez, "Clinical Issues in the Treatment of Chicano Male Gang Youth," *Hispanic Journal of Behavioral Sciences, 16*(1) (1994): 57–74.
46. J. D. Vigil, "Group Processes and Street Identity: Adolescent Chicano Gang Members," *Ethos, 16* (1988): 421–445; J. D. Vigil, "Street Socialization, Locura Behavior, and Violence Among Chicano Gang Members," in *Research Conference on Violence and Homicide in Hispanic Communities*, ed. J. F. Kraus, S. B. Sorenson, and P. D. Juarez (Los Angeles: UCLA Publication Services, 1988).

47. Belitz and Valdez, "Clinical Issues," p. 61.
48. Garcia Coll and others, "An Integrative Model."
49. J. Mercer, "In Defense of Racially and Culturally Non-Discriminatory Assessment," *School Psychology Review, 8* (1979): 89–115.
50. American Psychiatric Association, *Diagnostic and Statistical Manual of Mental Disorders,* 3rd ed. (Washington, D.C.: American Psychiatric Association, 1980).
51. J. J. Bauermeister and others, "Some Issues and Instruments for the Assessment of Attention-Deficit Hyperactivity Disorder in Puerto Rican Children," *Journal of Clinical Child Psychology, 19*(1) (1990): 9–16; American Psychiatric Association, *Diagnostic and Statistical Manual,* 4th ed.

Chapter Four

Intervening in Personal Contexts

You see, I left many friends back in elementary
I went to high school, they went to the penitentiary
PLACIDO VASQUEZ JR.

Although all young people have a number of similar concerns and experiences regarding self-concept, moral and existential questions, and intimate relationships, for Latino youth these concerns and experiences are influenced by face-to-face interactions in particular contexts. For example, a Latino youth's self-concept may be affected by prejudice on the part of teachers and classmates, reaction to his skin color on the part of his peers and even his own siblings, or reactions to his lack of fluency in the English language. In this chapter, we explore how contextual therapies may be employed to address selected problems unique to Latino youth that result from the interaction between culture and developmental processes in personal contexts such as family, school, and neighborhood.

We begin by exploring a contextual approach to assessment and suggesting ways of being responsive to culture. As we discussed in earlier chapters, the application of contextual therapies requires a different way of assessing "the problem." Next, we explore therapist-client interactions as a microsystemic context that relates to how the youth participates in his or her many social contexts. We then examine how solutions for particular problems should take into account the youth's participation in daily activity settings.

In other words, will the intervention create change in the social environments in which the youth lives? Existing versions of selected contextual interventions in current clinical practice are briefly examined for their applicability for working with Latino youth.

Defining the Youth's Problem

Most clinicians are guided in formulating interventions by the *referral problem,* which makes up the reason for the referral. The referral problem is often rooted in how the referral source (usually the parent, teacher, or social service agency) conceives of it. This initiates a culturally patterned process in which, in our society, the problem gradually becomes intrinsic to the person exhibiting it. In Chapter Two, we briefly discussed the positivist and historicist epistemologies that underlie most clinical practice and have long been established traditions in Western cultures.

From Referral to Presenting Problem to Diagnosis

As a result of the emphasis on the objectification of phenomena and on detached observation, the clinician shapes the referral problem into a *presenting problem,* which then becomes the basis for a diagnosis according to criteria established by the mental health system. But the process sometimes culminates in the client becoming the diagnosis—that is, taking it as part of his or her identity, such as, "Juanita is schizophrenic" or "José is ADHD" (has attention-deficit hyperactivity disorder).[1] In mainstream American society, many parents gratefully accept an expert's (the clinician's) diagnostic formulation because it fits their culturally determined view of the nature of personhood. In this view, a person engages in maladaptive behavior because of an intrinsic flaw, deficit, or disorder. The diagnosis reaffirms this view for both the parents and the youth. It is not uncommon to hear children attribute their difficulties at home or school to their diagnostic label. For example, Johnny might explain to his teacher that the reason he skips school is because of his school phobia, or Charlie may say that he is having a bad day in class because he did not take his Ritalin (to treat his ADHD).

Accepting this type of diagnostic formulation can be more difficult for many Latino parents. Although some problems may be viewed by some Latino parents as the result of "weak character" or inherited traits, Latino parents view many of the problems that bring Latino youth to the attention of mental health providers as temporary states that will resolve themselves with time and circumstance. One not infrequently employed solution is to send the youth with behavior problems to live with extended family members, who may reside in the country of origin. These kinds of solutions suggest that many Latino families take a contextual view to problems in living.

From a contextual perspective, the objectification of problem behavior into a diagnosis that focuses exclusively on the individual ignores how such behavior is multidetermined as well as affected by reciprocal interactions between the youth and observers (parents, teachers, diagnosticians, and so on). In other words, Thomas may be afraid to attend school because he has a low threshold for anxiety, has been increasingly teased by various classmates, and fears leaving home because he has repeatedly witnessed his father threatening his mother and wants to be there to protect her. Recognizing what Thomas is going through, his mother has allowed him to stay home on various occasions. But Thomas may be viewed by his teacher as a child who is overindulged and overprotected by his mother. The teacher responds by becoming emotionally distant and less responsive to Thomas, who then reacts with intense anxiety. The diagnostician sees Thomas at school in this heightened anxiety state and concludes that he suffers from an anxiety disorder, a school phobia.

Although contextual approaches to assessment are gaining in popularity, they are still not routinely used. Our contextual approach views the standard diagnostic process as typified by *transactions* responsive to situations and practices peculiar to our mental health delivery system, such as the requirement for DSM-IV diagnoses. We consider a diagnosis as a product of a series of reciprocal interactions among the diagnostician, the youth, the youth's family and persons in other immediate settings, and the referral source. From this vantage point, diagnoses are not static or immutable, and mental disorders arise from a lack of fit with the environment.[2]

Is Reduction of Symptoms Enough?

In Chapter Three, we discussed how a diagnostic system like the DSM objectifies the experience of the youth into an abstraction (the diagnosis), thus separating the phenomenology of the experience from the context of psychological intervention. For example, if a youth is given a diagnosis of major depression, the primary goal of therapy may be seen to be to reduce the symptoms. But does a reduction of symptoms constitute appropriate treatment? Is symptom reduction enough to make the life of a youth more meaningful and fulfilling? We wholeheartedly agree with Kirk J. Schneider that therapeutic outcome should be "gauged . . . by the broader textures and subtleties of real life experiences."[3]

Pepe, the ten-year-old boy we introduced in Chapter Three, was referred for treatment by the school and his parents because he was overly aggressive, impulsive, and extremely difficult to manage at home and at school. The description of the referral problem by Pepe's teachers and parents initiated a process that led to a set of diagnoses by an intake clinician at the children's psychiatric hospital where he was sent.

As we have often observed with immigrant Latino parents, the litany of Pepe's diagnoses had little meaning. Pepe's parents were much more concerned with how they could live in greater harmony with Pepe and their other children. Mother fondly recalled how, in El Salvador, Pepe had been "adopted" by the village in which they lived. Pepe had always been a very active child with a difficult temperament who required little sleep. Back in El Salvador, a neighbor who made very early deliveries in his horse-drawn cart to neighboring villages would take Pepe with him, often before the parents awakened. Pepe loved to go on these trips; he felt valued and important. Upon returning to the village, the neighbor, as much exhausted by his chores as by Pepe's high activity level and difficult temperament, would turn the child over to any one of a number of relatives and neighbors who would occupy his time while Mother tended to the younger children.

Upon coming to the United States, Pepe's parents joined a small Protestant church, whose members were largely Central American immigrants, with the expectation of finding the kind of closeness they had enjoyed in their native village. The church initially embraced the family but soon found Pepe too much to handle. The lack of acceptance of their child left the family feeling alienated and increasingly resentful of Pepe.

In Pepe's case, a contextual perspective requires that the clinician address the parents' framing of the problem; that is, how do we live in harmony with Pepe? In other words, how does Pepe's seizure disorder affect the way he relates to his family and his family to him? From this vantage point, the diagnosis is only important to the degree that it changes the negative environment or situations in the family, school, and neighborhood.

Therapist-Client Interaction

A youth's life and consequently his or her problems are interwoven in a number of activity settings in multiple contexts. From a contextual framework, the therapist must be prepared to intervene at multiple levels of contexts. This change in focus to multiple levels of intervention requires different skills and attitudes and a different conceptualization of the therapist role. The need to act on multiple levels of context brings culture into primacy in the therapy endeavor because, as Craig Smith, a narrative therapist, puts it, "The initial focus in therapy is on trying to grasp the local meanings and understandings of everyone involved, through creating a mutual, comfortable, and safe conversational environment."[4] Grasping the local meanings and understandings within the personal contexts of a youth—her family, for example—requires the therapist to delve into the culture of that youth and family.

Individual Therapy from a Contextual Perspective

For a contextual therapist, the therapist-client interaction is essential to positive outcomes and behavior change; it is the method by which one learns about the youth and continually makes adjustments to the therapy to bring about the desired change. At the microsystemic level, the unit of analysis in therapy is not just the youth-in-activity in different settings in face-to-face contexts such as family, school, and neighborhood but also the youth-in-interaction with the therapist in the therapy room, in the classroom (during school visits), or at home (during home visits)—the active, dramatic, live event in the context in which the therapist is observing and participating.[5] The reality addressed by the contextual therapist is that which is constructed by the *intersubjective* perspectives and experiences of the persons in the youth's microsystem.[6] The case of Salvador illustrates how perspectives from multiple observers provide a rich picture of who this youngster is.

> Salvador is a fourteen-year-old Guatemalan boy referred for outpatient therapy because of aggressive behavior and depression. His school counselor, the referral source, feels that Salvador is a very negative influence in the classroom; she sees him as a youngster striving to "stand out" as special and unique who is upset about his poor, disadvantaged status. His teachers see him as a mean-spirited, narcissistic, and manipulative youngster who has little empathy for his peers, who are mostly Mexican, Mexican American, and African American. Salvador's mother sees him as a caring son with a "short fuse," much like his deceased father. She feels bad that Salvador's father has died in the conflicts in their country, and that Salvador has come to the United States with her while his siblings remain with their grandparents. In his first therapy session, Salvador tells the therapist that, as bad as things were in his country when he came to the United States two years ago, he still hates being here. He describes how he and his mother now live in a dilapidated apartment complex in a neighborhood consisting of mostly Mexican and Cuban immigrants and African Americans. Youths from these three ethnic groups tease him, and he feels alienated both at school and in the neighborhood. He says that, if not for his mother, whom he feels he has to care for, he'd kill himself.

Each perspective—that of Salvador, his mother, his teachers, and the school counselor—help the therapist understand and appreciate the complexity of Salvador's dilemma. These perspectives and experiences help form the basis for a series of interventions on multiple levels, including individual therapy. Although individual therapy is informed by many of these perspectives and subsequent sets of information about Salvador in his various activity settings and contexts, it also adds a new context in which he can try out different behaviors, different ways of relating and interacting.

Contrasting Contextual Approaches to Individual Therapy

Narrative therapy approaches, which derive from a social constructionist perspective, operate in a contextual way. In our opinion,
narrative therapists see all individuals as microcosms of the world
around them. In this microcosm resides a universe of representations of and influences from past, present, and potential interactions with significant people in an individual's life in immediate
environments and in more remote contexts (for example, a rock
star with whom a youth identifies, or the sociopolitical values of the
nation in which a youth lives). In collaboration with the client, the
narrative therapist alters the client's life story by, for example,
"reauthoring" the client's identity. In emphasizing the need to perceive the world from the client's perspective through a collaboration with the client, the narrative therapist creates an opening into
both culture and development.

In contrast, *ecological* models of intervention consider the individual as a part of a system composed of a number of contexts
of increasing inclusiveness. A youth's activity settings are theaters
in which, as Richard L. Munger, an ecological psychologist describes it, "Certain activities flourish, others manage only to sur-
vive, and still others cannot even get started."[7] For the ecologically
oriented therapist, the therapy consists of working in and with the
environmental network in which the youth participates in order
to connect the youth with those activity settings in which desired
behavior changes can occur. Although one might envision how a
therapist might work at an individual level, the ecologically oriented therapist works with the individual-in-activity in larger contexts, that is, beyond the face-to-face interaction with the therapist.
Ecological interventions are discussed further in Chapters Five
through Eight.

Other individual therapies are also contextual in the way in
which they address culture. For example, a group from the Hispanic Research Center at Fordham University has described the effectiveness of an experimental intervention based on telling stories
about pictures depicting Latino cultural elements (like Latino
foods and games) and Latino families and neighborhoods in urban
settings.[8] This group has also developed an intervention called

Cuento Therapy, which depicts Latino role models and particularly targets the enhancement of ethnic identity in youth.[9] Kenneth J. Martinez and Diana M. Valdez have described a "transactional contextual model of play therapy" that specifically includes Latino elements (dolls, books, music, games, maps, and so on) that encourage the discussion of cultural issues.[10]

Family Therapy: From Limited Contextual Models to Ecological Models

The *family systems models* departed from traditional practice by viewing the identified patient as embedded in the family system. These therapies represent a major movement in psychology to propose a contextualist paradigm that significantly contrasts with therapies deriving from positivist and historicist perspectives. When first introduced, many of these family systems models retained strong elements of positivist models. As a result, some therapists, like Jill H. Freedman and Gene Combs, have criticized family systems theories because families are viewed as machines and therapists are considered independent of the influences of the families they are treating.[11] According to Freedman and Combs, these theories assumed that therapists could make "objective" assessments and were actually able to "fix" families.

Family therapy has evolved to become increasingly contextual. Some family therapists have become ecologists (such as José Szapocznik and Howard Liddle)[12] and some ecologically oriented psychologists (such as Scott Henggeler, Robert Friedman, and Richard Munger)[13] advocate the use of family systems therapy as one modality in an array of mental health services aimed at changing the activity settings within the environmental network in which the youth participates. These psychologists have extended the realm of possible interventions from the family to the community. Much as Roger Barker did in the 1960s,[14] today's social ecologists must learn to appreciate development and culture in order to intervene in a youth's activity settings and the various contexts in which these settings reside. One of the social ecologists' key contributions to contextual models is their shift from a focus on mental disorders or behavioral problems to an emphasis on environmental fit. Ecologists view an individual's problem as arising from poorness of fit between the individual's characteristics and needs and the environment, which is represented by the activity settings in which he or she participates in different levels of context. Some contextual therapists, like Szapocznik and his colleagues,[15] have described one-person family therapy aimed at changing family functioning; this hybrid modality merges individual therapy with family therapy within an ecological orientation. The focus in one-person family therapy is not on changing the individual but rather on changing a microsystem, the family.

Some family therapists expand the scope of their therapies when they incorporate culture into their practice. Braulio Montalvo and Manuel Gutierrez specifically addressed the cultural dimension in family therapy and drew attention to how culture can be used as a mask to deflect family problems.[16] Others have talked about how *triangulation* (an alliance of two family members against a third party) in family interactions cannot be understood outside of the family's cultural context.[17] Joseph M. Cervantes and Oscar Ramírez are among the few therapists who address mestizo spirituality—the result of the merging of Mexican Indian ideologies and European religious practices—in family therapy with Mexican Americans.[18] John Schwartzman even proposed that family therapy could be understood as an ethnography, the technique used in anthropology to study different cultures.[19] These therapists have brought greater attention to the need for mental health practitioners to examine the role of culture both in the presentation of "the problem" and in solutions to it.

A Shift in Role and Self-Perception of the Therapist

Although the social constructionist views the individual as a microcosm of the influences of the environment and the social ecologist views the individual with specific needs, desires, attitudes, and feelings in relation to a network of environmental influences, therapists from either persuasion have similar beliefs about how a therapist should interact with the client and family. It is important to examine these beliefs because they are crucial to working with Latino youth.

The Shift from Expert to Collaborator and Consultant

In contextual models, the therapist cannot assume an expert stance because it is antithetical to the underlying theory: what is important in the initial phase of therapy is to understand and appreciate the intricacies of the youth in activity settings in diverse contexts (for example, the youth's sense of himself as a gang member or as a gang member at home as opposed to in the neighborhood). It has been suggested that credibility is an important variable that must be considered in cultural techniques in therapy.[20] In our view, the therapist does not gain credibility because of who the therapist is, nor is credibility "achieved" by demonstration of expert knowledge. Rather, credibility is the product of understanding and appreciating youths in their various contexts, as they participate in activities that may or may not be rewarding, satisfying, and so on.

Narrative therapists talk about the importance of developing the ability to work within a "not knowing" stance. Ecologically oriented therapists talk about the need to develop the ability to collaborate and work in partnerships. Both talk about developing the ability in the therapist to learn from others, to learn together, and not to feel unduly challenged or defensive when questioned. They believe that if the client is not getting better, the service provider should either make alterations in the intervention or find alternative interventions rather than blame the client.

Shifting from Deficits to Strengths and Resources

Another important shift in contextual models is the focus on strengths and resources. At the microsystemic level, strengths and resources include those of the youth and the youth's family. The youth's strengths and resources can include biological and physical characteristics (height, physical attractiveness, health, athletic talent, temperament), cognitive abilities, emotional functioning, social skills, a positive ethnic identity, language fluencies, and biculturalism. Appreciation for a family's strengths and resources is also important and is too often ignored in noncontextual therapeutic interventions. These include the ability of the parents to provide age-appropriate monitoring and nurturance; household income; the physical and emotional health of the parents; social and community supports for the family; and the parents' education and employment, level of acculturation, ability to cope with acculturative stress, language fluencies, and so on. Contextual developmentalists like Bronfenbrenner and Brooks Gunn have emphasized the importance of attending to the interaction of the youth's physical, biological, and psychological attributes and the family's resources. But therapists are just beginning to heed their call. To work with Latino youth and their families, we believe that it is imperative to develop therapeutic interventions that directly attend to this interaction.

The Task of the Contextually Oriented Therapist

A main point of departure from traditional positivist and historicist methods is in their conceptualizations of mental health problems. When they take a contextualist view, therapists begin by carefully examining the unique characteristics of the person, face-to-face interactions that exacerbate or mitigate the problem in particular activity settings (for example, the neighborhood park where gang members hang out or the local Boy's and Girl's Club where other youths congregate), levels of contexts within which the problem occurs, and particular features of the time period in which the contexts are embedded (for example, a Cuban child entering the United States at the height of the Cuban missile crisis in the 1960s). We call this process *profiling* the youth-in-activity in context. This process results in a detailed description that we call a *lifescape*. Intervention is based on the notion that the expressed area of concern—or what most therapists often think of as the presenting problem—alerts the therapist to the poorness of fit between the youth and his environment. In practice, assessment and intervention are intertwined and continue simultaneously. The therapist is always assessing and making adjustments to interventions based on updated assessments.

Rather than imposing generalizations about culture, a contextual view examines culture from the perspective of the person or persons involved with one another in activities at different levels of context. Knowing, for example, that 80 percent of certain Latino youth value having straight hair and a lighter complexion may mislead us if a particular Dominican youth we are dealing with values

his dark skin color and kinky hair or gives these physical characteristics very different meanings. If we generalize about the value
of light skin color and straight hair, we might assume that this
youth also feels that way and erroneously base some of our interventions on that assumption. Or, realizing the pride this youth feels
in his skin color and kinky hair may lead us to pursue what has
happened in his particular development to result in such strong
ethnic identity as a Dominican and how we may sustain this asset
in his new environment. Generalizations may help guide assessment and intervention, but they must be corroborated by the experiences and perceptions of that particular youth.

A Case Example: Salvador

We now revisit the case of Salvador—the fourteen-year-old Guatemalan boy referred for outpatient therapy because of aggressive
behavior and depression—to illustrate our view of contextually oriented assessment and treatment.

Contextually Oriented Assessment at the Microsystemic Level

The contextually oriented therapist approaches the evaluative task
by collaborating with Salvador, his mother, and his teachers to find a
mutually agreed upon solution for Salvador's unfortunate predica-
ment of disliking the United States more than the war-torn country
he left. Together, they attempt to understand Salvador's problematic situation and the perceived area of concern from each interested party's viewpoint (in this case, Salvador's, the teacher's, the
parent's, and the therapist's) before attempting to solve it. Like an
ethnographer, the contextually oriented therapist approaches the
field of study (in this case, Salvador interacting at various activity
settings) without preconceived notions (for example, that Guatemalans are often passive, indirect in their communications, and
very sensitive to social hierarchies, or that North American teachers
often discriminate against Central Americans) that might influence the assessment process. The process of inquiry about the area
of concern is broached with Salvador, his mother, and his teachers
from a position of uncertainty. The therapist can only "know"
something from the particular perspective of Salvador or any of

the other participants in the activities in his contexts (at home or school). The focus of the assessment effort is to understand and appreciate where there is congruence or lack of congruence between Salvador and his daily activities in settings at each level of context. The purpose of the collaboration between the contextually oriented therapist, the youth who has been identified as having a problem, and the significant participants in that youth's contexts is to develop or optimize enduring interactions in contexts that are congruent with the youth's personal characteristics and attributes and his developmental needs.

As contextually oriented therapists, we might begin by profiling who Salvador is in terms of his physical, biological, and psychological characteristics and attributes. For example, Salvador is short, stocky, and dark-complected. He has been assessed with a Spanish version of one of the Wechsler scales of intelligence as performing in the upper fifth percentile of intelligence. His performance on the Spanish version of the Woodcock-Johnson battery of achievement tests was commensurate with his level of cognitive functioning. In addition, Salvador's temperament is characterized by high excitability, low tolerance to frustration (what his mother describes as a short fuse), and extroversion.

Next, we profile the perceptions that his teachers and his mother have of Salvador. His teachers have known him for only about three months, since he started high school. During a meeting with one of his teachers, the teacher tells the therapist that Salvador resembles most Central American students she has had. In her experience, they are easily influenced by negative peer groups because they so desperately want to fit in. She believes that Salvador is acting up in class to impress his peer group. She also thinks that his lack of empathy is the result of antisocial tendencies, which will eventually lead him into gangs, substance use, and increasing antisocial behavior and legal problems. Salvador was not assessed in the last year of middle school because, despite his very limited knowledge of English, he had a B average and did not call much attention to himself.

The teacher appears to perceive Salvador with her own generalizations from previous experience, and these generalizations have already cast a shroud of negative attributes on Salvador. The classrooms in the high school are very large, and the school's problems

with student-to-student and student-to-teacher violence are esca-
lating. One of Salvador's teachers was recently assaulted by an in-
halant-intoxicated Latino youth who resembles Salvador. Salvador
is more assertive and outgoing than most of the Central American
students his teachers have known and this increases their concerns.
His anger and despondency about his current situation are inter-
preted as indications of antisocial traits rather than a reaction to
an unfortunate set of circumstances.

Salvador's mother, Petrona, grew up in a small peasant village
in Guatemala. She looks Mayan and she speaks both Spanish and
Cachiquel, a Mayan language, but is semiliterate. She describes how
Salvador's father, José Luis, was a *ladino* (of European descent)
whom she met when he was a student at a Jesuit university in Guatemala City. He came to the village with a group of Jesuit priests, university students, and some Americans to speak about agrarian
rights of the villagers and provide assistance to those who had been
victimized by government troops. Petrona was fascinated by him.
He was sophisticated, worldly, idealistic, kind, and unlike any *ladino*
she had ever seen before. And unlike other *ladinos,* he did not ad-
here to the social hierarchy that created distance from the indigenous population. The two were married within a year, much to the
displeasure of Petrona's parents, who feared that this man was op-
portunistic, had "his head in the clouds," and was destined for trouble because of his "rabble-rousing."

After their marriage, José Luis and Petrona moved to Guatemala City while José Luis finished his studies. But even though fear
of violence dominated village life, she soon longed to go back to
the village because she felt so alienated in the city. She returned to
live with her parents and José Luis made frequent trips to be with
her while continuing his political activism and involvement with
the Jesuits. He fathered three children; Salvador was the first.

Petrona's parents' impressions proved to be partly true. During
a prolonged stay in the village eight years after their marriage, villagers found the body of José Luis, who had been brutally mur-
dered in the jungle, with a sign on his chest that read: *El Ladino
Pendejo* (The Foolish Ladino).

Salvador knows about the sign and what it said. He has been
very traumatized by his father's death, as well as by witnessing the
rampant violence and disappearances in the village. Petrona feels

a special bond with Salvador. *"¡Tiene los ojos de fuego de su papá!"* ("He has his father's fiery eyes!"), she once exclaimed, as tears streamed from her eyes. Where others saw Salvador as a Mayan Indian, his mother sees his *ladino* father in him. He has lived up to his mother's expectations. She describes him as a youth without a childhood, mature well beyond his age. He has his father's morals, sense of righteousness, and desire to fight for what is fair.

Petrona feels inadequate to deal with Salvador's teachers. She tells the therapist that she has had little schooling and can barely write in Spanish, even with all the efforts her now-deceased husband made to teach her. She says that Salvador is her "eyes, arms, and voice." She feels that in the United States people often dismiss her or see her as "too humble" *(muy humilde)*. As the therapist converses with her, he is struck by the emotional strength and courage of this woman, who has withstood the traumas in her life with so much dignity, serenity, wisdom, and optimism. She looks forward to next year when she feels she will be able to bring her other children and her parents to the United States with the help of a refugee organization in which she has become active.

Third, we might profile the face-to-face interactions and daily activities at the microsystemic level from Salvador's perspective. Additional assessment of Salvador reveals that he feels he does not fit in at school because of his poor fluency in English, his Mayan features, and his different values. *"Me ven como un pendejo"* ("They see me like a fool"), he angrily tells the evaluator. The word *pendejo* calls to mind the potential traumatizing link to his father. Salvador is quickly developing strong prejudices. He sees his Mexican and Mexican American peers as crude, vulgar, and cowardly, and African Americans as hostile and crass with no desire to learn. In his school in Guatemala, Salvador was "a star," a brilliant student admired by teachers and peers, a strong leader, and an excellent soccer player who was very popular with boys and girls alike. In this school, his Latino schoolmates have nicknamed him *Chango* (Monkey) because of his short stature, stocky build, and dark complexion. The concerns expressed by his teacher (his derisive treatment of his classmates, negative influence in the classroom, striving to stand out as special and unique, mean-spiritedness, and narcissism and lack of empathy) now begin to take on different meaning for the therapist. Salvador is yearning to re-create the school environment he had in

Guatemala. His expression of frustration is perceived by his teachers to reflect negative personal attributes. Unaware of his past history and the perceptions of others who know him, the teachers are at a considerable disadvantage in optimizing their interactions with Salvador and in providing rewarding activity settings for him in the school.

During classroom observations, the therapist notes how hard Salvador is trying to excel. On one occasion, Salvador is the first to raise his hand, is called on, and then proceeds to stumble with his English. Frustrated, his teacher tells him that if he did not know the answer he needed to let others answer. Salvador frowns, mutters something in Spanish, and receives a warning from the teacher about controlling his anger. At about that time, a Latino youngster next to his desk whispers: *"¡Chango salvaje, ooh, aah, ooh, aah!"* ("Wild monkey, ooh, aah, ooh, aah!"). Salvador fires off a vituperative and is quickly sent to the principal's office for failing to control his anger.

Contextually Oriented Intervention at the Microsystemic Level

In practice, it is difficult to separate interventions at each level of context because contexts are interwoven. In this section, we attempt to illustrate interventions at the microsystemic level.

Intervening at School

Following a series of meetings with teachers, mother, and Salvador, the therapist convenes a meeting with teachers and mother. Salvador agrees to a format in which the adults will meet first and then he will join the meeting later. The therapist asks each participant, starting with the mother, to describe what they see as the problem. The therapist translates for the mother with the assistance of one of the teachers who is also bilingual. With some guidance from the therapist, Petrona draws a picture of Salvador that casts him in the noble shadow of his father. One of the teachers remarks that she would never have guessed what Salvador has lived through. Gradually, comments from his teachers began to be peppered with observations of the boy's strengths and resources ("He is strong-willed and has a strong sense of fairness." "He has an intensity about him that makes other kids admire him." "He is excellent in math." "He seems very athletic."). Rather than see Petrona as an inadequate parent, the teachers begin to empathize with her and, equally important, to admire her. This is the beginning of an important collaboration to explore how Salvador could be provided with better opportunities to optimize his strengths and resources in various activity settings in the school. He qualified for the gifted program; but he does not meet the criteria for special education placement for an emotional disturbance. He is enrolled in the English-as-a-second-language program. His physical education teacher decides to talk to Salvador about trying out for the soccer team. One of the school counselors who is bilingual agrees to see Salvador once a week to talk about issues of acculturation, acculturative stresses, his efforts to fit in, and his tendency to lose his temper easily.

Salvador is then invited to join the meeting. Being particularly cognizant of Salvador's outgoing and outspoken nature, and knowing that he would not be easily intimidated in a meeting with so many adults, the therapist asks him to talk about what it was like for him at the beginning of his high school experience. The therapist is also cognizant that having his mother present will temper some of Salvador's emotional intensity and, bright as Salvador is, he will probably do very well in expressing himself in Spanish. Salvador proceeds to describe how things had been for him in Guatemala, and all can see how much pleasure this recollection brings to him. He next proceeds to describe what he had hoped for in his new school and how frustrated he feels at almost every turn.

The team presents its plans to address these concerns. Salvador at first appears unsure about how to take these suggestions and options. It appears that he is having difficulty accepting the notion that the school personnel has his best interests in mind. His only reluctance is in seeing the counselor, but his mother's gentle intervention—that she thinks this might be a good idea—leads him to say that he will try it. (Chapter Six will describe interventions that address linked contexts in greater detail.)

Intervening in the Family

In a separate meeting at the community mental health center, the therapist meets with Salvador and his mother. His mother explains that she is beginning to feel that she is losing her son. She feels that he is not accepting her authority as his mother and views her as not fully competent to manage the family affairs. She fears that she is losing his respect. Salvador gently protests that his mother does not know English and can barely read and write in Spanish. As he sees it, his mother cannot manage the family affairs without his help. What also emerges is that Salvador has difficulty seeing his mother in charge because in the village in Guatemala he had always considered his grandparents as the authority figures. He comments that his grandparents used to treat his mother like a young girl.

Petrona's difficulty in assuming a stronger parental role is further complicated by her perception of herself. She had lived most of her life in fear and had witnessed countless atrocities. In the United States, her fears and anxieties do not make much sense to Salvador and he is becoming increasingly upset at her for what he views as her helplessness. At one level, both her traumatization and that of Salvador illustrates what Linda Green, a cultural anthropologist, has called "the culture of fear." This ethos characterizes Guatemalan society and has its historical origins in the atrocities committed by the conquistadores during the Spanish invasion five hundred years ago.[21] Green comments that during her study in a small Guatemalan village, she was impressed by how often people used the saying: *"Lo mismo cuando se mato a Tecum Uman"* ("It is the same as when they killed Tecum Uman," a Mayan hero who died fighting the Spanish centuries ago).[22]

Then there is the issue of Salvador who, in Petrona's eyes, is her *ladino* son who daily reminds her of her husband. At one level, her relationship with her son plays out a very long history of a frustrating struggle: the efforts of the Indians to gain equal status with the Spanish. Salvador once describes that, in moments of desperation, his mother would mutter, "What do I know? I am but a poor Indian," to which Salvador would respond, "But I am not."

Salvador also was traumatized by the violence in Guatemala, but he wants to cut himself off emotionally from these experiences of the past. In so doing, he cannot see the link between his increasing irritability and his counterphobic reactions (being afraid of nothing and no one) and experiences in the Guatemalan village. He cannot see how he is disconnecting his feelings from his experiences.

Finally, there is the issue of spirituality. Petrona had been a devout Catholic in the village in Guatemala—going to church, praying the rosary frequently, and being very active in religious celebrations in the village. She misses the spirituality of her native village, which blended Indian and Spanish Catholic beliefs. She misses the feast days celebrated in the village. The Catholic church in her neighborhood in the United States cannot provide the function of reaffirming her connectedness with her new community, as did her village church, which had created and reaffirmed the social bonds within and between social classes (*ladinos* and peasants) in her village.

Goals of Therapy

Based on all of these assessments and interventions, family therapy might be directed toward several goals. First, Petrona needs to assume a position of parental authority and respect. The therapist might address Petrona's own perceptions of herself, which have thwarted her efforts to see herself as empowered and competent. He might ask her son how his mother's perceptions of herself have affected his views of her. In addition, his mother might be encouraged to enroll in a neighborhood parent-support group for recent immigrants that offers English classes in order to enhance further her sense of self-efficacy. Second, Petrona and Salvador need to recognize how each of them has been dealing with their traumatization in different ways, and how their traumatization is the result of recent and historical events. The therapist might direct attention to how each expresses his or her traumatization and how this expression affects the other. Third, Petrona needs to exercise her emerging parental authority once she begins to practice her parenting skills. The therapist might discuss with her and Salvador that there are certain tasks that his mother might undertake at home in order to practice these skills. Anticipating some resistance from Salvador, he might be provided with another activity setting (other than at home) to practice his leadership skills (for example, assuming a position of leadership in a youth church group or a club at school). Last, the therapist might explore the issue of spirituality. Knowing that Petrona feels a spiritual void, the therapist might suggest that Petrona inquire into a nearby church that shares more of her values, has a larger Latino congregation, and can offer a communitarian spirituality that provides an avenue for her to define herself in terms of that congregation (rather than in terms of the village in Guatemala).

The case of Salvador illustrates how a contextually oriented therapist might progress through the process of evaluation and therapy with particular attention to developmental and cultural aspects. We have emphasized how the process by which the therapist engages the youth, his parents, his teachers, and other adults in the youth's environment is as important as the substantive issues addressed in the interventions.

Conclusion

A contextual approach does not limit the type of intervention used. A specific therapy that is cognitive-behavioral may be used to treat a phobic child whereas a systems-oriented family therapy may be used to address how this same child has come to occupy a privileged status in the home. At the same time, a school intervention to develop a behavioral program to improve classroom participation might capitalize on the child's motivation to learn. As part of a contextual approach, these interventions are used to improve the environmental fit among any combination of activity settings and levels of context. In this sense, contextualism is more of a *metatheory* about how to intervene that can subsume other theories and still maintain its conceptual integrity. Chapters Five and Six examine linked contexts and will further illustrate the flexibility of contextually oriented interventions. Chapter Six describes the steps by which interventions are selected or developed.

Notes
1. S. Estroff, *Making It Crazy* (Berkeley: University of California Press, 1981).
2. R. L. Munger, "Ecological Trajectories in Child Mental Health," in *Innovative Approaches for Difficult-to-Treat Populations,* ed. S. W. Henggeler and A. B. Santos (Washington, D.C.: American Psychiatric Press, 1997).
3. K. J. Schneider, "Toward a Science of the Heart: Romanticism and Revival of Psychology," *American Psychologist, 53*(3) (1998): 277–289.

4. C. Smith, "Introduction: Comparing Traditional Therapies with Narrative Approaches," in *Narrative Therapies with Children and Adolescents,* ed. C. Smith and D. Nylund (New York: Guilford Press, 1997), 29.

5. In *World Hypotheses* (Berkeley: University of California Press, 1942), Stephen Pepper described contextualism using the root metaphor of the "dynamic, dramatic, active event," the historic event only as experienced in the here and now.

6. *Intersubjective* is a term used by Smith, "Comparing Traditional Therapies with Narrative Approaches."

7. Munger, "Ecological Trajectories," p. 17.

8. G. Costantino, R. G. Malgady, and L. H. Rogler, "Storytelling Through Pictures: Culturally Sensitive Psychotherapy for Hispanic Children and Adolescents," *Journal of Clinical Child Psychology, 23*(1) (1994): 13–20.

9. G. Costantino, R. G. Malgady, and L. H. Rogler, "Cuento Therapy: A Culturally Sensitive Modality for Puerto Rican Children," *Journal of Consulting and Clinical Psychology, 54*(5) (1986): 639–645.

10. K. J. Martinez and D. M. Valdez, "Cultural Considerations in Play Therapy with Hispanic Children," in *Working with Culture: Psychotherapeutic Interventions with Ethnic Minority Children and Adolescents,* ed. L. A. Vargas and J. D. Koss-Chioino (San Francisco: Jossey-Bass, 1992).

11. J. Freedman and G. Combs, *Narrative Therapy: The Social Construction of Preferred Realities* (New York: Norton, 1996).

12. J. Szapocznik and others, "The Evolution of Structural Ecosystemic Theory for Working with Latino Families," in *Psychological Interventions and Research with Latino Populations,* ed. J. G. Garcia and M. C. Zea (Needham Heights, Mass.: Allyn & Bacon, 1997); H. A. Liddle, "Conceptual and Clinical Dimensions of a Multidimensional, Multisystems Engagement Strategy in Family-Based Adolescent Treatment," *Psychotherapy, 32* (1995): 39–58.

13. S. W. Henggeler and C. M. Borduin, *Family Therapy and Beyond: A Multisystemic Approach to Treating the Behavior Problems of Children and Adolescents* (Pacific Grove, Calif.: Brooks/Cole, 1990); R. M. Friedman, K. Kutash, and A. J. Duchnowski, "The Population of Concern: Defining the Issues," in *Children's Mental Health: Creating Systems in a Changing Society,* ed. B. A. Stroul (Baltimore: Paul H. Brooks, 1996); R. M. Friedman, "Services and Service Delivery Systems for Children with Serious Emotional Disorders: Issues in Assessing Effectiveness," in *Evaluating Mental Health Services: How Do Programs for Children "Work" in the Real World?* ed. C. T. Nixon and D. A. Northrup (Thousand Oaks, Calif.: Sage, 1997); Munger, "Ecological Trajectories."

14. R. Barker, *Ecological Psychology: Concepts and Methods for Studying the Environment of Human Behavior* (Stanford, Calif.: Stanford University Press, 1968).

15. J. Szapocznik and W. M. Kurtines, *Breakthroughs in Family Therapy with Drug Abusing and Problem Youth* (New York: Springer, 1989); J. Szapocznik, W. M. Kurtines, A. Perez-Vidal, O. Hervis, and F. Foote, "One-Person Family Therapy," in *Handbook of Brief Psychotherapies*, ed. R. A. Wells and V. A. Gianetti (New York: Plenum, 1990).

16. B. Montalvo and M. Gutierrez, "A Perspective for the Use of the Cultural Dimension in Family Therapy," in *Cultural Perspectives in Family Therapy*, ed. C. J. Falicov (Gaithersburg, Md.: Aspen, 1983).

17. C. J. Falicov and L. Brudner-White, "The Shifting Family Triangle: The Issue of Cultural and Contextual Relativity," in *Cultural Perspectives in Family Therapy*, ed. C. J. Falicov (Gaithersburg, Md.: Aspen, 1983).

18. J. M. Cervantes and O. Ramírez, "Spirituality and Family Dynamics in Psychotherapy with Latino Children," in *Working with Culture: Psychotherapeutic Interventions with Ethnic Minority Children and Adolescents*, ed. L. A. Vargas and J. D. Koss-Chioino (San Francisco: Jossey-Bass, 1992).

19. J. Schwartzman, "Family Ethnography: A Tool for Clinicians," in *Cultural Perspectives in Family Therapy*, ed. C. J. Falicov (Gaithersburg, Md.: Aspen, 1983).

20. S. Sue and N. Zane, "The Role of Culture and Cultural Techniques in Psychotherapy: A Critique and Reformulation," *American Psychologist, 42* (1987): 37–45.

21. L. Green, "Fear as a Way of Life," *Cultural Anthropology: Journal of the Society for Cultural Anthropology, 9*(2) (1994): 227–256.

22. Green, "Fear as a Way of Life," pp. 235–236.

Chapter Five

Social Contexts
and Daily Activities

Kickback with my homies as the days roll by,
Puro East Side La Victoria *[gang] 'til the day I die.*
PLACIDO VASQUEZ JR.

In this chapter, we explore relationships between two or more social arenas that structure the activities of Latino children or adolescents—such as family and school, peer groups and family, family and street life (including gangs and drug use), and family and sexual partners. In Chapter Two these contexts were described as part of the *mesosystem,* referring to the social ecology of linked, face-to-face settings.[1] By way of introduction, we first review the frequently discussed concept of *risk,* which guides so many studies, and suggest ways in which it might be adapted to a contextual approach. The more recent concept of *environmental fit* is then briefly reviewed as a theoretical tool that enhances a contextual approach to interventions. We discuss these concepts because of their relevance to adolescent development, a subject to which a large part of this chapter is devoted. This discussion is followed by an exploration of how culture and development together affect the normal activities and situations of Latino children and adolescents, and the nature of the problems these youths may experience.

Relationships between the family and the school shape youths' activities ("daily practices") and youths in turn influence both their activities and their experiences of home and school. These intersecting chains of relationships directly affect school success or failure. For example, when a youth loses interest and "ditches" school (is truant), is expelled, or drops out, these actions could be attributed in part to learning disabilities or cognitive deficits. But whether a biopsychological cause is or is not implicated, aspects of the relationships between the youth, the youth's family, and the school are always germane to the problem and its potential solution.[2]

It is also important to highlight that children's development is affected by cultural guidelines that influence how their parents and other socializing agents assess and value life choices toward the goal of maximizing those behaviors that make their children most acceptable in their eyes. One writer phrases it as those "socialization goals that teach the strategies necessary for survival."[3]

Understanding how face-to-face interactions influence development in linked social contexts is central to clinical work that takes a contextual approach. Juan's story, recalled in the following section, illustrates how his development is influenced by the traditional pattern of relationships in his immigrant family; the juvenile justice system and its response to deviant behavior, drug use, and gang membership; and early adolescent sexual experience and fatherhood.

> Juan, a sixteen-year-old who was born in Mexico, is seen for follow-up during house arrest for his second felony (possession of a quantity of methamphetamine). He tells his therapist that his ex-girlfriend recently revealed that he was the father of her four-month-old daughter. Although the therapist is privately dismayed on hearing this news, Juan expresses delight at the prospect of having a child, once his paternity has been established in court. For her part, Juan's mother expresses her eagerness to bring this grandchild into her already large household, and appears to accept fully this added responsibility. Although the therapist thinks about the potential stresses and strains of this event for Juan and his mother, they in turn are pointing out the strong resemblance between the new baby and Juan's niece's infant picture, both of whose photographs are proudly displayed on a shelf in the living room. Juan's mother then comments on how Juan's house arrest had been a positive experience, because he has acquired child-care skills, having taken charge of his eighteen-month-old niece while her mother is at work. The mother worries, however, that Juan takes too many risks when he gets restless and sometimes leaves the house at night, despite continuing surprise checks by the probation officers.

The expectations of the therapist in this case do not always parallel those of Juan or his mother. What they see as a positive event in Juan's development—fathering a child—is usually seen as risky teenage behavior by health care and mental health care providers. For Juan's mother, it indicates that Juan has matured and is ready to assume family responsibilities. (There are a number of reports of Latino youth who "mature" out of gang and delinquent activities by having a family.) Her definition of positive development is oriented by standards appropriate to rural life and minimal demands for higher education. In contrast, the mental health care provider's standards are tied to the economy of postindustrial societies and the expectation that youths will attain the qualifications to obtain dependable and well-remunerated jobs to support new families. Teenage pregnancy is risky behavior because mainstream American society views it as an unwelcome economic and social burden, assuming that adolescents will not be able to fulfill familial responsibilities adequately.

Concepts of Risk and Development

A consideration of linked social contexts is highly relevant to the transition from childhood to adolescence, when youths focus on activities beyond their homes and schools and are more involved with developing their selves and social identities. This and the following section discuss two social science concepts—risk and environmental fit—that offer ways to understand these important development processes. The widespread double view of human development (that is, observer versus subject) is nowhere more salient than in the concept of risk, which fuels endless analyses of the causes of child and adolescent behavior problems. From an epidemiological perspective, a condition of risk can predict the emergence or presence of behaviors considered disruptive or deviant. A corresponding notion is that of *multiple-risk families,* which refers to the adverse conditions that some families experience. In one longitudinal study of families in which one or both parents had a diagnosed psychiatric disorder, the family environment was described as "chaotic" and "extremely stressed," and the children assessed as "at high risk."[4] However, some children were identified as "resilient" because they did not have a psychiatric diagnosis and were functioning successfully as rated on a number of measures. The investigators concluded that children who were troubled early in their lives and were labeled as more vulnerable suffered more distress and problem behaviors during their early adolescent years.

The difficulty in approaching youths' problems using a risk model is that causality is attributed to characteristics internal to the youth and separate from the situations and activities in which development takes place. The investigators in the longitudinal study cited in the preceding paragraph explored constitutional variables—health, intelligence, temperament, and self-perceptions—comparing resilient children with troubled children along these dimensions.[5] They also attended to relationships with peers, relatives in the home, and related households. However, the limitation of their approach was that they used information on these relationships to measure the extent and impact of youths' troubles rather than viewing relationships as central to daily practices on which interventions might be based. In Juan's case, for example, these investigators would take into consideration as risk factors his relationship with his girlfriend, the subsequent birth of a child to a fourteen-year-old mother and a sixteen-year-old father, his drug use, and the house arrest for his second felony.

A contextual approach would instead take a perspective that focuses on the family's value system—which supports fatherhood for youths; confers higher, adult status on Juan; and affords Juan a greater measure of self-esteem. A contextualized interpretation of his situation might be construed as a therapeutic opportunity to suggest to Juan that his new responsibilities and satisfactions are important to his family and his role in it. Given the importance of family to Juan and his stated desire to please his mother, a therapist could suggest to Juan ways in which his new role and its activities might adequately substitute for the self-enhancement provided by gang membership and its socially deviant activities.

An approach to development through exploring social context has been suggested by Michael Rutter and his colleagues, who move toward a contextual view of risk.[6] Their formulation focuses on transactions between people and environments, examining individual differences in environmental exposure to risk. It does not include culture as a conceptual tool, but it does attend to certain aspects of culture, such as ethnicity and racial discrimination. Although perpetuating an individualistic approach to studying the causes of problems in development, they focus on a broad range of environmental factors—such as geography, social networks, and income and job opportunities—in addition to past experiences and personal responses. Rutter and his colleagues lump these factors together, however, rather than sorting them into meaningful levels of social experience (contexts) within particular patterns of relationships at specific times during the life span.

From a clinical perspective the concept of risk can be said to pertain to researchers' notions about the source of problems rather than reflecting ways in which the risk takers themselves think about their behavior and the meanings associated with their life situations. Cynthia Lightfoot takes the latter perspective in accounting for risk behavior.[7] Her approach is contextual to the extent that it includes consideration of how development proceeds as a reciprocal interaction between youths and the social settings that frame and structure their activities. Based on in-depth interviews with adolescents, she concluded that risk taking is a "basic social psychological process" manifest in children's play and a way for adolescents to establish and maintain a social identity.[8] Risk-taking behavior can in fact be seen as heroic activity for youths, central to the creative construction of their life stories and to efforts to shape their self-identities. However, it is also the case that much risky behavior that is defined as heroic has the peer group as its audience.

Unfortunately, the behaviors that many organized adolescent peer groups espouse are considered socially deviant by adults; the judgment of deviance is part of a sociocultural context. Although many youths in the United States identify with the violent but charmed lives of heroes such as Rambo or the Terminator, most Latino parents either have no knowledge of these media figures or simply cannot understand them because they are outside the range of their experience. Traditional culture heroes—such as Emilio Zapata for Mexicans or César Chávez for Mexican Americans—have practically disappeared for present-day youths. In our opinion as clinicians, the salient question that must be addressed in order to understand (or intervene in) adolescent development is a transformation of the usual question, "With whom is the child or youth most identified?" Instead, it is, "With whom is the youth most actively engaged in daily life practices?" or "With whom does the youth interact most meaningfully as he or she develops?"

Risk and Ritual

Anthropologists are fond of describing how tribal societies provide culturally patterned ritual opportunities for pubescent youth to create a heroic identity for themselves. These rituals have been labeled "rites of passage"[9] and are noted for the seemingly nefarious ways in which the transition to adult status is fraught with danger and difficult trials. The obvious point is that small, nonindustrialized societies rarely left the risk taking and process of self-identification to the control of the youths themselves. These societies were often mired in internecine warfare, providing hero-warrior roles for young (postpubertal) men, and difficult family situations for postmenarchial young women, in which they were tested for their caretaking, homemaking, and food-getting abilities.

Many Latinos in the United States maintain some customary rites of passage. A young woman's fifteenth birthday (*la quinceañera*) is celebrated as a community recognition of her eligibility for marriage as well as her moral responsibility to delay marriage and sexual activity until family approval is forthcoming. Young men of fifteen are awarded freedom to be away from home, on their own without explanation—behavior earlier denied them by more traditional authoritarian parents. In a rural setting, these culturally patterned situations appear to have been appropriate tests of moral and social responsibility for youth. However, in more complex urban settings teeming with challenges from the dominant youth culture and a well-established ethnic street culture, the traditional tests seem to lack significance for many Latino youths. In turn, the youths usually create their own initiation experiences that attempt to deal with the transition to adulthood in an intellectually challenging and often dangerous environment at school and on the streets. The heroic patterns for these transitional experiences are frequently borrowed from folk themes presented in the mass-media entertainment world, which are laden with violence, sexuality, and disregard for humanitarian values.

Ronald Gallimore and his colleagues report on how immigrant parents in California, aware of the complexities related to urban life in this country and the need to protect their children, restrict their freedom of movement to the circle of relatives or neighborhood friends.[10] A longitudinal study of Mexican and Central American families followed children from age five to middle-school age. The study found that these middle-school youths showed few signs of oppositional behavior in early adolescence. Using an *ecocultural theory* as described by Thomas Weisner,[11] the researchers examined the families' daily activities, which were partly constructed by the families themselves and partly determined by the broader social systems in which the families were involved in the United States, such as jobs, churches, and so on. As is usually the case among immigrant families, parents—often single mothers—spent long hours at work. Yet despite their parents' absence, many of the early adolescent children actively participated with their parents in supporting and structuring after-school activities that restricted their social lives to close-to-home settings. Rather than oppose their parents' values and regulations, these youths supported their values and beliefs about the preferred family environment and their own relationship within it. In this population, three different types of parenting resulted in differential school success among the children. One group of parents openly restricted their daughters' friendships and activities. Their daughters continued to be involved in school but were not among the high achievers. A second group of parents permitted their children to exercise control over some aspects of their lives, making choices and decisions within approved frameworks. These parents monitored all aspects of their children's lives. The children of these parents were most successful in school and many were high achievers. In a third group of families, parents were generally permissive and did not overly attempt to structure and limit their children's choices of activities when it came to friends, school, or street life. This was especially the case for boys, who were generally unsuccessful in school because their unfettered sense of self-determination led to choices that ignored schoolwork and attendance.

The situations of the immigrant families described imply that risk-taking behavior is perhaps not an elemental psychological process that expresses itself in the same way in all youths. Definitions of what young people find challenging and the extent to which they collaborate in arranging their activities with parents or teachers depend on who has the greatest impact on the youths' lives and who influences their decisions. Important aspects of each situation include the nature and organization of the youth's family within particular sociocultural contexts (social class, income levels, neighborhoods) as well family traditions. They also include encounters with mentors (often serendipitous), who may have a significant impact on a youth's life. Do certain families (or other contexts) buffer the deleterious effects of destructive peer groups, or do some families learn how to prepare their growing children to understand the challenges of life on the street and respond to them in ways that protect them from negative effects?

Environmental Fit

A final notion we wish to discuss is that of environmental fit.[12] This idea seeks to explain why adolescence (especially in the early years) can be a time of turbulence for so many youths by implicating the social environment rather than frequently cited biopsychological factors such as changes in hormone levels, effects of rapid growth, or accelerated cognitive development. It proposes that negative psychological effects can occur when there is a mismatch between the needs of adolescents and the ways in which their social environments are structured. The sites of most daily activities—home and school—are assessed in relation to their needs and very often found to be developmentally inappropriate. Transition to middle school, for example, poses a number of difficulties. Middle schools are larger than elementary schools and subject students to more controls and fewer opportunities for decision making and self-management at a time when most adolescents are beginning to seek out opportunities for greater autonomy. These and other failures of the school environment to meet developmental needs are exacerbated by the lack of systematic ways to take individual needs into account or by failure to orient instruction and activities toward the different levels of maturation of individual children. The failure to assist students with learning or behavior problems during this sensitive and fast-changing period can negatively affect students' self-esteem in numerous ways. The effect of this neglect was low motivation and eventually school failure for Glorisa, a sixteen-year-old Mexican American girl.

> Glorisa had continuous problems with school that became particularly serious after she entered sixth grade. On finding out that Glorisa's father was an alcoholic who physically and verbally abused his wife and other members of the family, her school counselor referred her for family therapy. During the assessment interview Glorisa admitted to having a hard time understanding school assignments. That year she had failed both math and history. She confessed

that she constantly worried about her future and did not know what she was going to do. Shortly after this interview, an aunt who had studied to become a beautician suggested that this might also be good idea for Glorisa, who immediately decided that she was interested in beauty school. When seen on follow-up a year later Glorisa was happy in her beautician training program and was performing at a passing level in school. Her attitude toward school and life had radically changed and she was looking forward to her senior year.

The family setting can also be examined from the perspective of environmental fit. A mismatch is relatively easy to spot when parents become increasingly authoritarian and controlling in response to their children asserting needs for separation and independence, and when they fail to negotiate ways in which their children can be independent at least some of the time. This was the case with Maria, fifteen years old, whose rebelliousness accelerated when her parents became more restrictive.

Maria's parents had emigrated from Mexico when she was only two years old. She was a special-education student doing fairly well at school, quiet and respectful with her parents and teachers. Her relationships with peers at school were often problematic, however, and she was suspended for possession of marijuana after being found with a new friend in the girls' bathroom rolling a joint. Her parents accepted her claim of innocence but kept her at home most of the time. Then one day she became actively interested in a boyfriend. On hearing about this, her parents responded by keeping her at home as much as possible. They allowed the boyfriend to visit when Maria was chaperoned. But Maria began to let her boyfriend into the house after her parents had gone to bed. After discovering the two kissing in her bedroom late one night, the furious parents banned her relationship with the boy and ordered her confined to the home during all after-school hours. Maria responded by sneaking out of her bedroom window at night to meet the boyfriend, which angered her parents into imposing even more restrictions, arousing in Maria an intense and openly expressed attitude of resentment and conflict.

Sociocultural context can have an important influence on how parents direct their children's activities outside of the home. Immigrant parents often view their primary goal to be to protect their children from the dangers of violent neighborhoods. The idea of a mismatch between a youth's needs and environments could be extended to the usual situation that all ethnic cultures are in dynamic relationships with dominant-culture institutions and thus are in an ongoing situation of cultural discontinuity. This notion has been proposed to account for problem behaviors among youths such as gang membership and oppositional behavior at school. The idea has been reframed recently as the inability of many students to manage discontinuities between their disparate worlds (different sociocultural contexts).[13]

The California research group led by Ronald Gallimore advocates a balanced view of the situation of immigrant families by examining cultural continuities as well as discontinuities, such as immigrant parents' placing high value on education for their offspring.[14] The capacity of a child or adolescent to make the transition between multiple worlds (different sociocultural contexts)—perhaps speaking Spanish at home, English at school, and Caló (a street dialect) with peers, each language possessing different patterns of affect and meaning—may be key to understanding the genesis and continuation of a youth's behavior problems. We suggest that understanding how youths navigate boundaries and manage their diverse worlds at home, on the streets and in school, offers a fruitful avenue for interventions. This subject will be explored in the next chapter. In this chapter, the studies and cases we present describe ways in which boundaries between worlds can become difficult to cross as adolescent development proceeds from middle school through high school.

Developmental Contexts: Family and School

A large literature addresses the problems of underachievement and dropout rates among Latino children and adolescents. The most recent census figures for Latinos age twenty-five and over show that 53.1 percent of males and females have completed four years of high school, and 10.3 percent of males and 8.3 percent of females have completed four years of college.[15] These figures gain more meaning when compared with white males and females, of whom 82.7 percent have completed high school and 24.3 percent have completed college. These significant differences call for an explanation that goes beyond differences in income. Furthermore, although the overall rates have improved steadily over the years since 1970, there are still significant differences in school completion among youth from different Latino cultures: fewer Mexicans complete high school, whereas the numbers of Puerto Ricans and Cubans are almost equal in this category. But there are greater differences among those finishing four years of college: only 6.5 percent of Mexicans do compared with 11.0 percent of Puerto Ricans and 18.8 percent of Cubans. Clearly, there are different situations affecting educational opportunities and performance in different Latino communities in the United States.

In this section we discuss the relationship between family and school performance in terms of the settings and activities that affect this relationship. We also explore how peer relationships may mediate family influences in affecting both school performance and behavior problems that can lead to dropping out or simply to an inadequate education.

Parenting Practices and School Success

Four types of parents have been identified: *authoritarian parents, authoritative parents, indulgent parents,* and *neglectful parents.*[16] Authoritarian parents are strict, high in control and coerciveness but relatively low in warmth, and little involved in their children's activities. They are more likely to make unilateral decisions on behalf of their children. Authoritative parents are firm but warm, very involved in their children's lives, and engage in joint decision making. They maintain consistent household routines. Indulgent parents are high in warmth but exert little control over their children. They allow their children considerable autonomy and leeway in decision making. Neglectful parents are neither particularly warm nor involved in their children's activities; they are lax in their supervision and do not provide consistent household routines.[17]

It has been widely suggested that differences in parenting practices affect school performance—specifically, authoritative parenting (parental acceptance, supervision and strictness, and autonomy or agency granting) results in healthy psychological development and school success.[18] Latino families socialize their offspring to value education and their parenting style is most frequently described as authoritarian, emphasizing obedience and conformity. However, this description may not reflect the reality of parenting practices across Latino cultures. In our observations, those parents who are high in control and demand obedience can also be affectionate and indulgent with material goods. Furthermore, this view fails to take the temporal dimension of development into account in at least two ways. Younger children are indulged more frequently than older children. And many immigrant parents view the age of fifteen as the threshold of adulthood; at that time, gender differences become more important. They then treat their sons and daughters in very different ways. Sons are released into the world and expected to be responsible adults, whereas daughters are subjected to more intense supervision to protect the honor of the family, as the value placed on virginity before marriage is high.

Many parents, having had little education themselves and feeling intimidated by school tasks, cannot provide daily support for scholastic endeavors.[19] It has been noted that the educational level of Mexican and Mexican American mothers is positively correlated with the use of questions and praise in teaching their children.[20] Moreover, mothers with less education use more modeling, which involves less interaction with their children, than do mothers with more education. One study asserts that low-income Latino parents *do* have the interest and ability to become involved in their children's academic pursuits but may need specific direction from teachers.[21]

Immigrant Parents and School

A number of issues are related to the school experiences of immigrant families and their children. One of the most important is that of language. When parents speak Spanish at home (and the majority of Latinos do so), their contacts with the school can be unsatisfactory unless they are also fluent in English or the school provides bilingual personnel. Moreover, these contacts can cause embarrassment to the children. Low socioeconomic status further contributes to lack of communication between parents and teachers and other school functionaries, because the parents feel socially inferior. Many immigrant youth or children of immigrants wish to blend in with their English-speaking peers and selectively dissociate themselves from their parents as well as those more recently arrived.

In family therapy, Ernesto, an eleven-year-old Salvadoran, insists on respond-ing to his therapist in English even though the therapist is conducting the ses-sion in Spanish. His father teases him that he is becoming too American for the family, which leads Ernesto to roll his eyes and his siblings to giggle. An-gered, his parents complain that Ernesto feels he is too good for the family and they resent his increasing sense of entitlement. Ernesto responds that his par-ents are too old-fashioned and unaware of what is "in" or "cool." He and his siblings feel ashamed of their parents, especially when they attempt to speak English to their children's teachers. Ernesto's sixteen-year-old brother, who often serves as the interpreter for his parents, laments in English that the teachers think their parents are backward or, worse yet, "dumb." Understand-ing the gist of what his older son is telling the therapist, Ernesto's father tells the therapist apologetically: *"Es que somos del campo."* ("It's because we are country people.")

Many Central American families, such as those from Guate-mala, El Salvador, and Nicaragua, are not just immigrants but also refugees from war-torn communities. The relationship between these families and the educational system is often quite different from that of other immigrants.[22] Most youths, some of whom are sent to the United States to avoid conscription into the army or other dangers, live with relatives or even alone. They are highly motivated to achieve in school to justify the sacrifices their parents made in order for them to receive the opportunities of U.S. soci-ety. They work hard to assist parents to come here or to adjust to life here. They often take on part-time jobs and still maintain good averages in their schoolwork. Ernesto's older brother is a good illus-tration of this—he helps his parents interface with the English-speaking world and is also a high achiever. This boy's motivation is associated with feelings of love, caring, and family closeness, es-pecially toward his parents.

In contrast, some immigrant youths can become quite anxious because they fear their career plans will not be realized. This was expressed in a focus group made up of eighth-grade students, all recent Mexican immigrants, who were discussing issues around lan-guage. Although all of the students supported the idea of being bilingual, one expressed her concern: "We will never be able to learn English well enough in four years to get into college" (our translation).

Educational Success and Failure in Latino Youth

Although parents across Latino cultural groups generally agree on the high value of education, many of their children harbor deep doubts that completing a high school education will reward them with better job opportunities and higher incomes. The issue of adolescent achievement motivation is frequently discussed in the literature in attempts to explain the school failures of the involuntary Latino immigrants, including Mexican Americans and second-generation Puerto Ricans. We need to raise the question of whether the problem lies within the individual youth or in the daily practices to which he or she is exposed. What are the most significant reasons for educational success or failure?

A number of observers advance the notion that cultural conflicts between home and school values and patterns of social behavior in the larger society are key to understanding the lack of academic success among Mexican Americans and second-generation Puerto Rican youth (the latter often referred to as *Neo Ricans* or *Nuyoricans*).[23] But how are these conflicts constituted? There is the subtle, discriminatory effect of the way Latino cultural groups (in particular, the involuntary Latinos or unmeltable ethnics, who are described further in Chapter One) are socially categorized into a castelike social status based on the assumption that the groups' members are incapable of achieving careers in the white-collar or professional arenas.[24] Another factor is that of inaccuracies in the definition of educational competencies and their relationship to the cultural, social, and economic realities of Latinos. As noted in Chapter Three, the analysis of "failure" as the result of either genetic or cultural deficits in Latino youths arises out of what John Ogbu has described as a "decontextualization of competencies" (based on his analysis of African American youth).[25] Latino youths strongly internalize the value of being intimately integrated within their primary social groups, their family of origin, their extended family, and their immediate neighborhood. Many if not most Latino children aspire to better lives and to "greatness," primarily to honor their families and reward their parents. This motivation frequently serves to inhibit valuing and using individualistic competitive behavior to succeed in scholastic and career endeavors.

Perhaps the most important factor in school failure is the frequently subtle—but also at times blatant—discrimination that

Latino youths experience in school. The story of Melba illustrates not only the impact of discrimination by her teachers on her academic career but also the complexities of these events when influenced by interactions with her family, thus demonstrating the effect on her development of relationships between different social contexts.

> Three years after a course of family therapy, Melba, twenty-one years old, was enrolled in a community college. When we talked recently, Melba was planning to finish her A.A. degree and take a third and fourth year at the local university to earn a B.A. degree.

> Melba recalled how in high school she had experienced serious conflict with her Spanish teacher. Melba suffers from anxiety and depression and was often restless and disobedient in high school, talking to a friend during class, answering back to teachers, and ditching school after a night of heavy drinking. Of Mexican descent, her mother had been born and raised in the United States and had not taught Spanish to her daughter. The Spanish language teacher seemed to dislike Melba for her oppositional behavior and was annoyed by her restlessness in class. She often embarrassed Melba in front of the other students because she felt that Melba should be more knowledgeable about and interested in Spanish. One day, after chastising her for talking in class, she told Melba to go to the principal's office. Melba shouted back at her in a fit of anger and acute embarrassment. Shaking with fear before the principal and in tears, she was given the choice of dropping all language classes or being expelled from school. She was told that she was a poor student and unsuited for higher education. Despite her deep desire to attain a college degree, Melba took this incident to heart, became pregnant shortly thereafter, and dropped out of school.

> However, Melba's mother believed in her abilities and supported her ambitions. She assisted Melba in getting a graduate equivalency diploma (G.E.D.) and helped with the baby so that Melba could take college courses on a part-time basis while working to support her child. With encouragement from her family and psychological treatment to help her manage her moods (she had individual, short-term counseling following twelve sessions of family therapy), Melba became a successful student.

Nonimmigrant families have much higher expectations of the school system than do immigrant families, but these expectations are often tempered by earlier experiences with discrimination. This can lead to alienation from the school system that further defeats its capacity to involve parents in assisting failing students.[26] Further, the experiences of youth are often synergistic with those of their parents. Maria Eugenia Matute-Bianchi describes how many Latino youths in California reject schooling as an avenue to achieve the occupational and class status to which they aspire.[27] The youths report that their parents would not object to their dropping out of school.

A study in Miami compared Chicano, Puerto Rican, and Cuban students who drop out of school. It listed factors to account for leaving school, including recency of migration, educational plans related to parents' expectations, and rejection of educational goals and values. This study also examined the contributions of socioeconomic status, gender, and accelerated role transitions to dropping out of school.[28] Higher socioeconomic status and two-parent households are highly correlated with fewer dropouts among Cuban youth, as compared to other Latino groups, in which the association is not as strong. Studies that look at parental education and occupation as predictors of achievement among Mexican American students offer mixed conclusions.[29] Among Chicanos and Puerto Ricans in Miami, being female increases the odds of dropping out; in contrast, being male is reported as significant for the dropout rate of Mexican American youth in the Southwest and California. We will discuss the importance of other factors, specifically relationships among family, gender, and the impact of accelerated role transitions, later in this chapter.

The Situations of Families and Peers

Peer group influence expands as a child matures, finally becoming extremely important in middle to late adolescence.[30] We propose that children encounter a world of meanings, and through negotiation with other persons contribute to shaping their own developmental experiences as participants in shared cultural activities. Because both settings and activities are patterned by culture, the relative importance of parents versus peers and the content of developmental activities, such as parenting practices and peer group relationships, varies according to culturally patterned situations. Despite abundant sources of variation, there seems to be a universal process in which children appropriate or interpret knowledge that results in the formation of autonomous peer subcultures that have at least one primary goal: gaining control over adult authority. Other common goals are friendship and intimacy as well as social differentiation based on age and gender roles, and later in development on other markers, such as social class, "race," and ethnicity. Early adolescents also use peers to help them deal with confusion, fears, and conflicts.[31]

Among Latinos, different situations in the various cultures represented in the United States are contextual to this process and lead to differences in how families and peer groups relate to each other in the contest for influence over youths. For example, situations are shaped by whether the family is from an involuntary or a voluntary ethnic group or is a family of refugees, which in turn relates to the educational level of parents, their economic opportunities, and the presence or absence of traditional family patterns. Unfortunately, very few studies report on positive daily relationships between the family and a youth's peer group. Most studies of Latino children and adolescents explore the topic of families and peers in order to explain behavior problems—drug use, gang membership and behavior, teen pregnancy, dropout rates, and aggression. A frequent conclusion is that authoritative parenting consisting of acceptance and involvement along with strictness and supervision can protect against problem behavior in adolescence. However, we propose that psychological interventions require an in-depth understanding of relationships among youth, families, peer involvement, and activities.

Impact on Delinquency

A number of studies of non-Latino youth have shown that poor parental monitoring can have a significant influence on adolescent delinquency and drug use as well as on academic achievement.[32] As mentioned earlier, many Latino parents seem to lose the ability to monitor their children closely, especially their sons, after they turn fifteen, when the youths are informally granted adult status because they are reproductively mature. (They are, however, still far from being "productively mature," that is, able to earn a living in a technologically advanced urban setting.) How this pattern interacts with findings on the positive influence on adolescent adjustment of authoritative parenting is not known. However, the finding by Laurence Steinberg and colleagues that peer group influence was more significant for Hispanic adolescents, fourteen to eighteen years old, in Wisconsin and Northern California (Latino culture unspecified), was not related in their study to immigrant status or differential acculturation between parents and children.

What the studies of Steinberg and his colleagues make very clear is the role that parents unconsciously play in slotting their children toward particular peer groups by fostering particular traits.[33] Peers select their companions based on similar behavior and reputation. The investigators conclude that "parenting practices predict adolescent personality traits and orientations" and these in turn predict the type of peer group in which their child will be involved.[34] This effect held across ethnic groups, including the Latino group. Given the often-repeated finding that peer drug use is the most significant predictor of individual drug use and delinquency, it is important to ask two questions: What family patterns are conducive to traits that lead to participation in problem behavior peer groups? And do these patterns differ among Latino cultures?

In a study in Rochester, New York, of Hispanic seventh- and eighth-grade students (Latino culture unspecified), investigators found that single-parent families and parents who were less involved with their adolescent children predicted delinquent behavior.[35] On the positive side, however, attachment to family was associated with the perception of strong family involvement, which has an indirect protective effect against delinquency. Single-parent families and parents who had low involvement with children were not associated with delinquency among white and African American youths, confirming the investigators' observations that family plays a more important role in the lives of Latino adolescents. A likely explanation is that single mothers are too preoccupied with earning a living for their families, and perhaps also with caring for young children, to devote enough attention to their adolescent children.

Socioeconomic disadvantage has been implicated as an important influence on behavior problems in youth, regardless of ethnicity. Vonnie McLloyd documents how "harsh, inconsistent parenting" and exposure to chronic stressors mediate the relationship between poverty and "children's socio-emotional functioning."[36] Carefully designed research, controlling for maternal IQ, maternal education, and other maternal characteristics, found significant effects of poverty on children's verbal and cognitive skills. Certain Latino groups—immigrant Mexican, Central American, and many Puerto Rican families—live at the poverty level. Moreover, because of high fertility rates, Latino children (especially those of immigrants) are overrepresented in the national population (14 percent of all children in 1992). Continuous poverty has an additional effect: from a contextual perspective, low-income neighborhoods seem to be characterized by more aggression and acting out in children, perhaps the result of peer-group influence and lower-quality schools and child-care facilities or of parents feeling that their children need to learn to defend themselves in neighborhoods where crime is frequent.[37] Considering the importance of peer influence on drug use, the ready availability of aggressive, delinquent friends means that there are also more and earlier opportunities for using drugs. Recent studies show that the earlier the exposure to drugs (both legal and illicit), the more likely that delinquent behavior initiated in early adolescence (symptoms of conduct disorder, in particular) will continue into young adulthood.[38]

Latino Gangs

The general public seems to have little in-depth information on Latino adolescent gangs and some misconceptions about them, in part because of the fear and discomfort the topic inspires. Moreover, the popular media rarely portray gangs from the perspective of the gang members themselves.

Gangs on the West Coast were established some decades ago, following a general trend in the United States of youths in immigrant, socially marginal communities. Most Latino males by mid-adolescence participate in a territorial pattern of peer group relationships (called *klikas* in Southern California and parts of the Southwest) within their neighborhoods (or *barrios*).[39] The traditional name for peer cohorts in Mexico is *palomilla*—equivalent to *close friends* or *comrades*—a normative type of friendship. Such groups do not usually exhibit antisocial behavior. The name given to peer cohorts in California, and synonymously to those active in street culture, is *cholos,* a term borrowed from some Latin American cultures that denotes a mixture of European and indigenous cultures and peoples. It is interesting as an ethnic folk label that highlights the cultural mixture integral to Latino cultures and also transitional (and marginal) social status. The gang is a special type of peer group, one that fills many diverse needs, from ethnic-identity formation to surrogate family to social expression of anger and rebellion.

In Latin America, extended families are very frequently localized in urban barrios, villages, and small towns. One's closest peers are also near or distant cousins, so parents exercise authority over all the youth in the barrio. The pattern of relatives living nearby continues in the United States, and at times it can have both negative and positive outcomes. Whereas relatives can provide much-needed support for stressed, low-income immigrant families, in some cases residential proximity can also enhance the effect of dysfunctional family patterns, such as overuse or abuse of alcohol or drugs by uncles and aunts and older cousins. In addition, a legacy of gang membership may be continued by a few male relatives, who serve as role models as tough, macho survivors. These cousins or uncles may provide protection in violent neighborhoods, where there is also a supply of early adolescent or younger boys—"wannabes"—who are attracted to street life by the *veteranos* or older gang members. Veteranos sometimes are over thirty years old with families of their own, yet still actively engaged in a gang. It must be emphasized strongly that most Mexican American youth attracted to gangs (as well as Puerto Rican gang members) spend only a few years in the gang and give up antisocial acting out and drug use by late adolescence. Many mature out of this street life when they form families of their own, even if doing so is the result of getting a teenaged *novia* (girlfriend) pregnant and assuming the father role without actually setting up a household with her.

Gang careers among early adolescents or preadolescents usually begin with hanging out with older boys, who set them on a course of petty thievery or give them jobs as messengers and lookouts. The first *klikas* that appear in a barrio neighborhood are made up of males, twelve to fifteen years old. After a difficult initiation of physical pummeling or even dangerous ordeals—such as doing a "drive by"—boys take on different roles: some may carry out petty criminal acts on their own but interact with gang members for parties, athletic games, and "bull" sessions; others participate in very serious deviant activities as suppliers of drugs, drug addicts (*tecatos*), and burglars or muggers. A small number (referred to as *psychos* or *vatos locos*) adopt a crazy and even violent bravado, exhibiting extreme antisocial behavior that often incites other members to defend their desire for "respect" when another group encroaches on their territory or activities.

Research on gangs provides rather confusing information on the relationship between Latino ethnicity and gang involvement. Joan Moore and Diego Vigil assert that Chicano youth gangs do not promote crime but help with normal adolescent concerns of security, respect, and approval from peers, and offer gender role identification and support.[40] However, many gangs encourage deviant and sometimes violent behavior, a potent expression of the rage, anger, and rebelliousness manifested by some youths who have serious problems. As noted earlier and discussed briefly in Chapter Three, Vigil shows how gangs serve a number of psychological needs, especially managing the identity crisis, frequently offering street-culture role models when none are available at home. The outward trappings of this process of personal and social identification are the insignia of the gang—special clothes, signs, tattoos, names, expressions, and so on. In addition, there is the need for a sense of belonging and to be respected in a society that confers low status and prestige on poor, uneducated foreigners, whether immigrants or involuntary ethnic persons. As also mentioned in Chapter Three, the importance of "respect" as an element in all relationships is a central—one might say basic—tenet of Latino cultures. Angry adolescents will tell you that they have been "dissed" (disrespected) as a justification for some violent act on their part.

Families and Gangs

The situation for Mexican Americans and immigrant Mexican youth appears to be much the same when it comes to gang behavior as it is for Puerto Rican gang members in the barrios of New

York and elsewhere.[41] Although the focus of Philippe Bourgois's book is on cocaine dealing and substance abuse among young adults as an expression of social marginality in Spanish Harlem, he shows clearly how street culture and aspects of family life are related. At one point his protagonist, Primo, says, "You see it was me and my older cousins. I was a little nigga' and they was already thieving. . . . When I was like ten that was my first one."[42] But the reason Primo gives for his entry into street crime is a strong desire for what he calls "little things"—new sneakers, a radio, a comic book. And although Primo's mother repeatedly harangues him for stealing and staying out at night, he knows that her income as a single parent does not stretch to meet the needs of all of her children. As a "man" (at ten years of age when he began stealing) he feels he has to get the money for himself.

In a study in East Los Angeles, Peter Adler and his colleagues conclude that families of gang members are more likely to have mothers born in Mexico who speak only Spanish, violence in the family, few family joint activities, little ability of parents to transmit emotional support, and little supervision of children.[43] These investigators suggest that this type of family life is based in social ecology, caused by the stresses and poverty that immigrants experience in urban settings. However, our research in two southwestern states shows that immigrant Mexican families generally have fewer negative characteristics, including violence, abusive relationships, and desertion by fathers. Immigrant parents in our clinical samples are more frequently still together, and family life is less chaotic than that of the Mexican Americans in these same groups despite social environmental stresses.

Using reports from incarcerated gang and non-gang Latino youths (specific culture and region unspecified), Jean-Marie Lyon, Scott Henggeler, and James Hall found similar patterns of family relations among the two groups, as well as similar peer relations across Caucasian and Hispanic gangs.[44] What then are the salient factors that influence antisocial and delinquent behavior? Based on this study, as well as on the descriptive studies by Diego Vigil and Joan Moore in Los Angeles, gang membership or immigrant status alone does not sufficiently account for either criminal activities or drug use.

Girl Gangs

Girl gangs are also found in many Latino communities.[45] Their territorial notions and activities do not differ very much from that of male gangs, but there is less frequent deviant behavior, especially violence and drug use. Like the young men, these young women are motivated by identity concerns. In Puerto Rican girl gangs, the decision to search for self as a gang member has been described as arising from rejection of popular social identities related to class, race, and gender. Girl gang members reject traditional Latin culture for "modern" North American lifeways. The ideas espoused by the girls include a form of feminism that rejects passivity, subordination, and dependence on males. There is considerable emphasis on sexual mores, and gang rules mandate only one sexual partner at a time in an attempt to avoid "cheap" behavior—that is, behavior like that of prostitutes. Using intravenous drugs such as heroin and cocaine is not considered acceptable, whereas using alcohol and marijuana and dealing these drugs is routine. This same attitude applies to petty crime. Early sexual experience is the norm and, as will be further discussed in the following section, pregnancy by the age of fifteen is not uncommon.

The phenomenon of gangs differs with sociocultural context at different periods in history. Bryan Page presents an interesting argument to explain the disappearance of Cuban gangs in Miami by showing how increasing prosperity and social dominance in the Cuban community made gangs irrelevant.[46] Page's study further illustrates the value of an ecological perspective in which deviant behavior is viewed largely as a response to adverse social and economic situations.

Drug Use and Families

Family life has been directly associated with drug use in adolescents as affected by parental drug use patterns, the child's perception of parental attitudes toward drug use, and life in single-parent (mother-headed) households. Investigators in Miami questioned Mexican, Puerto Rican, and Cuban adolescents and found that both Puerto Rican and Mexican youths living in female-headed

...olds had higher rates of drinking, drug use, and risky be-
...avior when compared with Cubans.[47] For Puerto Rican youth in
particular, family structure does seem to affect overall problem
behavior—defined here as the quantity of alcohol and drugs used
and frequency of drinking in the past month. For Cuban youth
family structure appears to be unrelated to high levels of alcohol
and drug use. Although there are gender differences in the extent
of risk-taking behavior among Mexicans and Puerto Ricans, with
males reporting higher rates of drug use, both are affected by single-parent households in similar ways. These findings suggest,
again, the importance of the economic and other difficulties that
single mothers experience; Cuban mothers have better economic
opportunities. This study also found that Spanish language use predicted lower rates of substance use for both Cuban and Mexican
youths, suggesting that lower rates of acculturation to North American behavior patterns may be protective.

In a study of Mexican American adolescent children of alco-
holics in the Southwest, Manuel Barrera and his colleagues found
a positive association between parental alcoholism and life stress
in their children as well as between psychological symptoms and
rates of alcohol use in adolescents.[48] But compared with Caucasian
youth, Mexican American youth show less vulnerability to the stress
associated with alcoholic parents. The authors speculate that this
may be explained by as-yet unidentified cultural factors, perhaps
related to parenting or to personal characteristics contributing to
resiliency in these Mexican American youth.

In a contextual approach, it is the relationships among such
factors—parenting practices and youth's responses, for example—
that need to be observed in order to understand why certain
youths are more or less stressed.

Families, Peers, and Sexuality

There is much discussion in the popular media and scholarly literature, as well as among health care professionals and social-ser-
vice providers, that although Latina adolescents are less likely than
other groups to be sexually active at an early age, they are also
much less likely to use contraception or to have an abortion once
pregnant.[49] As a result, the national birth rate for Latina teens over

fifteen years is twice that of non-Latina whites; for those fifteen years or younger, the birth rate is four times as high. However, more of these teenage births occur in married couples as compared with other ethnic groups. This reflects the widespread expectation that a Latino youth who fathers a child should marry the mother. There is a view that reproductive maturity is as important a marker of adulthood as productive maturity. Attitudes toward motherhood and fatherhood are very positive, as illustrated by Juan (described earlier), who is sixteen and in trouble with the law, yet eager to assume the father role. There is little doubt that although most parents are initially dismayed at the prospect of their teenage child having a child, once born this child is fully accepted as another family member to be cared for and loved. Indeed, Mexican and Mexican American teenagers in the Southwest seem to look on the event as a normal rite of passage into adult status even if they do not marry or remain with the parent of their child. For girls, pregnancy appears to parallel the risk-taking behavior of boys, a quasi-planned self-scheduling of the transition to adulthood.

A dark underside to the intimacy and interdependence of Latino family life can be associated with immoral and deviant sexuality. Single male relatives living with the family of a brother or sister will sometimes use younger cousins, nieces, or nephews as sexual objects. An intense sense of shame and a common taboo against talking about sex with one's elders (considered highly disrespectful in many families) conspire to keep the abuse secret. Maria, whose story of parental restriction and growing resentment appeared earlier in this chapter, suffered some special problems.

> Maria's parents' obsession with protecting her from sexual experience, although not unusual in traditional Latino families, is exacerbated by Maria's having been raped repeatedly at the age of ten by a cousin who was seven years older. The boy had been taken in by her family and was a favorite nephew of her father. Perhaps for this reason, or because of fear, shame, or guilt, Maria did not tell her parents until more than two years after the rapes happened. Maria appears depressed when she tells us that the rape experience takes over her feelings and thoughts daily so that she cannot concentrate in school. Mother apparently has not been very helpful because, although she has filed a complaint with the police, she tells the therapist that she finds it hard to face what has happened and does not believe in revenge. Father also offers little

help to Maria because he fears hearing about the details. He is caught up in intense feelings of shame over his failure to protect his daughter, not just from abusive experience but, according to tradition, from all sexual experience prior to marriage. That the youth who sexually abused his daughter is a nephew who lived in his home at the time of the abuse makes the truth almost unbearable. For the therapist, it helps explain the father's ready anger and obsessiveness about Maria.

Gender, Sexuality, and Risky Behavior

When we saw Maria a year after family therapy ended, she had broken up with her boyfriend, who had left her infected with chlamydia. Even with medication, Maria complained of continuing pain, and her mother seemed more anxious and distraught than during the last visit six months earlier. However, the mother had finally sought treatment for depression and was taking medication. Somewhat ironically, at our last visit Maria's parents appeared more accepting of her boyfriend. Furthermore, Maria seemed less in conflict with her father. He had changed his work schedule and was at home during the evenings so that he could spend more time with her.

In Maria's case, the value placed on an early but continuous relationship with a *novio* (boyfriend or fiancé) is evident. However, this kind of exclusivity does not always extend to the male partner, who may have other girlfriends on the side. As noted for girl gang members, both peers and families censure young women who have more than one partner at a time, which is considered loose behavior. Yet the double standard is alive and well among many males of all ages in Latino cultures, even though traditions in many families insist on fidelity in part because of religious values.

It is apparent that the traditional pattern of gender relationships is being eroded by acculturation to North American norms. A study in Detroit of Hispanic youth (specific culture not identified) found that more highly acculturated women were more likely to have had more than one sexual partner in the last year, to have had oral and anal sex, to have had experience with non-Latino partners, and to have used condoms. (This study group ranged in age from fifteen to twenty-four and does not reliably reflect adolescent behavior. However, it suggests that the direction of change may be through sexual relationships as youths adopt a North American pattern of dating contrary to Latino cultural norms.)[50] The implications for the spread of sexually transmitted diseases, including HIV infection, are both positive (more condom use) and negative (more sexual partners and more risky sexual practices). The high rates of HIV and other sexually transmitted diseases (STDs) reported for Latino adolescents are considered to be the result of earlier sexual activity. A national survey showed that 33 percent of Latino males aged fifteen have had sexual intercourse.[51] An important aspect of the problem is gender role behavior. Can a young woman refuse to have sex or insist that her partner use a condom? This course of action involves a sense of self-efficacy when confronted with an onslaught of pressure both from a boy to satisfy his sexual desires and from one's own sexual arousal. Yet many and perhaps most Latinas learn very early that their gender role includes a mandate to please males. Rick Zimmerman and his colleagues found few quantifiable differences among tenth-grade adolescents in three ethnic groups (including Hispanics in Miami) in the ability to refuse unwanted sex. However, more young Hispanic women than white women beyond adolescence reported that they found it more difficult to say no.[52] A positive attitude toward early sexual activity and considering peers to be important predicted less ability to say no to unwanted sex among all youth, regardless of ethnic group. Again, the important role of the family in a youth's activities is highlighted. A balance between family and peer group influence is essential if the family is cohesive enough to demonstrate and support values and activities that are conducive to the youth having fewer developmental problems, such as being able to avoid unwanted sex.

Conclusion

In Chapter Two we made the observation that therapies focused on the individual limit the range of interventions because they ignore the fact that development and culture are interwoven within identifiable social contexts. Here we add that there are also very practical reasons to broaden interventions beyond those modalities that include only a youth and a therapist. A common problem in individual psychological interventions is that they do not generalize to many important life contexts of the child or adolescent.

A child or adolescent in treatment may report relief from distressing feelings or a lessening of socially deviant ways of seeing the world or behaving. But with the passing of time the difficulties and problem behaviors that first drew the youth into therapy frequently reappear. Given the linkages between the developmental contexts described in this chapter, it seems obvious that even contextual family therapies may fall short of the goal of restoring or re-creating a healthy developmental path.

Notes

1. U. Bronfenbrenner, "Ecological Systems Theory," in *Annals of Child Development*, vol. 6, *Six Theories of Child Development*, ed. R. Vasta (Greenwich, Conn.: JAI Press, 1989).

2. R. M. Lerner, J. V. Lerner, and J. Tubman, "Organismic and Contextual Cases for Development in Adolescence: A Developmental Contextual View," in *Biology of Adolescent Behavior and Development*, ed. G. R. Adams, R. Montemayer, and T. P. Gullotta (Thousand Oaks, Calif.: Sage, 1989), 11–37.

3. L. H. Zayas and F. Solari, "Early Childhood Socialization in Hispanic Families: Context, Culture, and Practice Implications," *Professional Psychology: Research and Practice*, 25 (1994): 201.

4. M. Radke-Yarrow and E. Brown, "Resilience and Vulnerability in Children of Multiple-Risk Families," *Development and Psychopathology*, 5 (1993): 581–592.

5. Radke-Yarrow and Brown, "Resilience and Vulnerability."

6. M. Rutter, L. Champion, D. Quinton, B. Maughan, and A. Pickles, "Understanding Individual Differences in Environmental Risk Exposure," in *Examining Lives in Context*, ed. P. Moen, G. Elder Jr., and K. Luscher (Washington, D.C.: American Psychological Association Press, 1995), 61–95.

7. C. Lightfoot, *The Culture of Adolescent Risk-Taking* (New York: Guilford Press, 1997).

8. Lightfoot, *The Culture of Adolescent Risk-Taking*, p. 157.

9. R. L. Munroe and R. H. Munroe, *Cross-Cultural Human Development*, Life-Span Human Development Series (Pacific Grove, Calif.: Brooks/Cole, 1975); A. van Gennep, *The Rites of Passage* (New York: Routledge, 1960 [first published in 1908]).

10. L. Reese, K. Kroesen, and R. Gallimore, "Agency and School Performance Among Urban Latino Youth," paper presented at the annual meeting of the American Educational Research Association, Chicago (Mar. 1997); K. Kroesen, L. Reese, and R. Gallimore, "Navigating

Multiple Worlds: Latino Children Becoming Adolescents in Los Angeles," paper presented at the annual meeting of the American Anthropological Association, Washington, D.C. (Nov. 1997).

11. T. S. Weisner, "Ecocultural Niches of Early Childhood: A Cross-Cultural Perspective," in *Development During Middle Childhood: The Years from Six to Twelve*, ed. W. A. Collins (Washington D.C.: National Academy Press, 1984).

12. J.S.C. Eccles and others, "Development During Adolescence: The Impact of Stage-Environment Fit on Young Adolescents' Experiences in Schools and Families," *American Psychologist, 48*(2) (1993): 90–101.

13. P. Phelan, A. L. Davison, and H. C. Yu, *Adolescents' Worlds: Negotiating Family, Peers and School* (New York: Teachers College Press, 1998).

14. Reese, Kroesen, and Gallimore, "Agency and School Performance"; Kroesen, Reese, and Gallimore, "Navigating Multiple Worlds."

15. U.S. Bureau of the Census, *U.S. Census of Population, U.S. Summary*, PC80–1-C1, and *Current Population Reports;* and unpublished data.

16. E. Maccoby and J. Martin, "Socialization in the Context of the Family: Parent-Child Interaction," in *Handbook of Child Psychology*, vol. 4, *Socialization, Personality, and Child Development*, 4th ed., series ed. P. H. Mussen, vol. ed. E. M. Hetherington (New York: Wiley, 1983), 1–101.

17. L. Steinberg, S. M. Dornbusch, and B. Bradford Brown, "Ethnic Differences in Adolescent Achievement: An Ecological Perspective," *American Psychologist* (June 1992): 723–728.

18. Reese, Kroesen, and Gallimore, "Agency and School Performance"; Kroesen, Reese, and Gallimore, "Navigating Multiple Worlds."

19. C. Goldenberg and R. Gallimore, "Local Knowledge, Research Knowledge, and Educational Change: A Case Study of First-Grade Spanish-Reading Improvement," *Educational Researcher, 20*(8) (1991): 2–14.

20. L. M. Laosa and R. W. Henderson, "Cognitive Socialization and Competence: The Academic Development of Chicanos," in *Chicano School Failure and Success: Research and Policy Agendas for the 1990s*, ed. R. R. Valencia (Bristol, Pa.: Falmer Press, 1991), 164–199.

21. R. Gallimore, C. N. Goldenberg, and T. S. Weisner, "The Social Construction of Subjective Reality in Activity Settings: Implications for Community Psychology," *American Journal of Community Psychology, 21*(4) (1993): 537–559.

22. M. M. Suarez-Orozco, *Central American Refugees and U.S. High Schools: A Psychosocial Study of Motivation and Achievement* (Stanford, Calif.: Stanford University Press, 1989).

23. Gallimore, Goldenberg, and Weisner, "The Social Construction of Subjective Reality"; Reese, Kroesen, and Gallimore, "Agency and School Performance."

24. H. T. Trueba, "From Failure to Success: The Roles of Culture and Cultural Conflict in the Academic Achievement of Chicano Students," in *Chicano School Failure and Success: Research and Policy Agendas for the 1990s,* ed. R. R. Valencia (Bristol, Pa.: Falmer Press, 1991), 151–163.

25. J. U. Ogbu, "A Cultural Ecology of Competence Among Inner-City Blacks," in *Beginnings: The Social and Affective Development of Black Children,* ed. M. B. Spencer, G. K. Brookins, and W. R. Allen (Hillsdale, N.J.: Erlbaum, 1985).

26. H. Romo, *Improving Ethnic and Racial Relations in the Schools* (Charleston, W. Va.: ERIC Clearinghouse on Rural Education and Small Schools, 1997).

27. M. E. Matute-Bianchi, "Ethnic Identities and Patterns of School Success and Failure Among Mexican-Descent and Japanese American Students in a California High School: An Ethnographic Analysis," *American Journal of Education* (Nov. 1986): 233–255.

28. W. Velez, "High School Attrition Among Hispanic and Non-Hispanic White Youths," *Sociology of Education, 62* (1989): 119–133.

29. F. D. Bean and M. Tienda, *The Hispanic Population of the United States* (New York: Russell Sage Foundation, 1987).

30. W. A. Corsaro and D. Eder, "Children's Peer Cultures," *Annual Review of Sociology, 16* (1990): 197–220.

31. Corsaro and Eder, "Children's Peer Cultures."

32. R. Loeber and T. Dishion, "Early Predictors of Male Adolescent Delinquency: A Review," *Psychological Bulletin, 94* (1983): 68–99; R. H. Coombs and J. Landsverk, "Parenting Styles and Substance Use During Childhood and Adolescence," *Journal of Marriage and the Family, 50* (1988): 473–482.

33. L. Steinberg, N. E. Darling, and A. C. Fletcher in collaboration with B. B. Brown and S. M. Dornbusch, "Authoritative Parenting and Adolescent Adjustment: An Ecological Journey," in *Examining Lives in Context,* ed. P. Moen, G. Elder Jr., and K. Luscher (Washington, D.C.: American Psychological Association Press, 1995), 423–466.

34. Steinberg, Darling, and Fletcher, "Authoritative Parenting."

35. C. Smith and M. D. Krohn, "Delinquency and Family Life Among Male Adolescents: The Role of Ethnicity," *Journal of Youth and Adolescence, 24*(1) (1995): 69–93. A study in Miami found a direct relationship between reported family support and decreased use of drugs among eighth-grade students in Little Havana; see S. Frauenglass, D. K. Routh, H. M. Pantin, and C. A. Mason, "Family Support Decreases Influences of Deviant Peers on Hispanic Adolescents' Substance Use," *Journal of Clinical Child Psychology, 26* (1997): 15–23.

36. V. C. McLloyd, "Socioeconomic Disadvantage and Child Development," *American Psychologist, 53*(2) (1998): 185–204.

37. *Consequences of Growing Up Poor,* ed. G. Duncan and J. Brooks-Gunn (New York: Russell Sage Foundation, 1997).

38. J. Brooks, "Adolescent Drug Abuse and Co-Occurring Behavior Problems," presentation at the National Meeting of the American Society of Addiction Medicine, New Orleans (Apr. 16–19, 1998).

39. Information on Mexican American gangs can be found in J. D. Vigil, *Barrio Gangs: Street Life and Identity in Southern California* (University of Texas Press: Austin, 1988); J. Moore and others, *Homeboys: Gang, Drugs, Prison in the Barrios of Los Angeles* (Philadelphia: Temple University Press, 1978); and R. Horowitz, *Honor and the American Dream: Culture and Identity in a Chicano Community* (New Jersey: Rutgers University Press, 1983). Perspectives based on the authors' research and clinical experience in two southwestern cities have also been included.

40. J. W. Moore and J. D. Vigil, "Chicano Gangs: Group Norms and Individual Factors Related to Adult Criminality," *Atzlàn, 18* (1989): 27–44.

41. P. Bourgois, *In Search of Respect: Selling Crack in the Barrio* (New York: Cambridge University Press, 1996), 195.

42. Bourgois, *In Search of Respect,* pp. 196–197.

43. P. Adler, C. Ovando, and D. Hocevar, "Familiar Correlates of Gang Membership: An Exploratory Study of Mexican-American Youth," *Hispanic Journal of Behavioral Sciences, 6* (1984): 65–76.

44. J. Lyon, S. Henggeler, and J. A. Hall, "The Family Relations, Peer Relations, and Criminal Activities of Caucasian and Hispanic-American Gang Members," *Journal of Abnormal Child Psychology, 20* (1992): 439–447.

45. A. Campbell, "Self-Definition by Rejection," *Social Problems, 34* (1987): 451–466; J. C. Quicker, *Homegirls: Characterizing Chicana Gangs* (Madison, Conn.: International Universities Press, 1984); R. Horowitz, *Honor and the American Dream* (Chicago: University of Chicago Press, 1983).

46. J. B. Page, "Vulcans and Jutes: Cuban Fraternities and Their Disappearance," *Free Inquiry, 25* (special issue no. 2, 1997): 65–73.

47. D. McDermott, "The Relationship of Parental Drug Use to Adolescent Drug Use," *Adolescence, XIX* (spring 1984): 89–97; and R. H. Coombs, M. J. Paulson, and M. A. Richardson, "Peer vs. Parental Influence in Substance Use Among Hispanic and Anglo Children and Adolescents," *Journal of Youth and Adolescence, 20* (1991): 73–87, summarize the range of psychosocial factors that have been reported to influence substance use among children and adolescents, many of which are mentioned in this chapter.

48. M. Barrera Jr., S. A. Li, and L. Chassin, "Ethnic Group Differences in Vulnerability to Parental Alcoholism and Life Stress: A Study of Hispanic and Non-Hispanic Caucasian Adolescents," *American Journal of Community Psychology, 21* (1993): 15–35.

49. P. I. Erickson, "Contraceptive Methods: Do Hispanic Adolescents and Their Family Planning Care Providers Think About Contraceptive Methods in the Same Way?" *Medical Anthropology, 17* (1997): 65–82.

50. K. Ford and A. E. Norris, "Urban Hispanic Adolescents and Young Adults: Relationship of Acculturation to Sexual Behavior," *Journal of Sex Research, 30*(4) (1993): 316–323.

51. B. Van Oss Marín and C. A. Gomez, "Latino Culture and Sex: Implications for HIV Prevention," in *Psychological Interventions and Research with Latino Populations,* ed. J. G. Garcia and M. C. Zea (Needham Heights, Mass.: Allyn & Bacon, 1997), 73–93.

52. R. S. Zimmerman, S. Sprecher, L. Langer, and C. D. Holloway, "Adolescents' Perceived Ability to Say 'No' to Unwanted Sex," *Journal of Adolescent Research* (July 1995): 383–399.

Chapter Six

Intervening in Linked Contexts

To a facility, just another casualty,
We ain't a gang, we're a crazy-ass family.
PLACIDO VASQUEZ JR.

In Chapters Three and Four, we explained why the paradigms on which most therapeutic interventions are based might have a limited range of therapeutic effects. Many widely used interventions are designed to focus exclusively or primarily on individual youths rather than on their relationships within the social contexts in which their development takes place.[1] From a contextual perspective, a youth's distressful experiences arise from behavioral and emotional responses to problematic situations associated with different life arenas. Recall Juan (whom we presented in Chapter Five) and his stealing, alcoholic binges, using and perhaps dealing illicit drugs, long-term conflict with his younger sister, and oppositional behavior with his parents: all are associated in different ways with various social contexts—family, school, peers, and the local juvenile justice system. In addition, now that Juan is embracing single fatherhood with its complex responsibilities and arrangements, these contexts will change, and new contexts will become important foci for intervening in Juan's problems.

From a contextual perspective, there is no reason to evaluate a particular environment as good or bad, desirable or nondesirable. We do not mean to suggest that some environments might not have more negative influences on a youth's development than others. However, evaluating the environment per se does not guide us in developing or selecting appropriate or efficacious interventions. A salient concept that might better guide the formulation of interventions is *lack of fit* with an environment, or as one author puts it, the *congruence* and *incongruence* between the youth's activities, developmental needs, and contexts.[2]

Alan E. Kazdin describes the relevance of the "scope of impairment" and suggests that multiple problems often relate to the same developmental processes.[3] Both Juan's rebelliousness at home and his close bond with his fellow gang members serve his need to be autonomous and his desire to achieve a satisfying personal and social identity. We agree with Kazdin when he emphasizes that the task of treatment goes beyond dealing with symptom presentation. Initially, assessment should include profiling those aspects of social contexts related to a distressed youth's problematic behavior. In the case of Juan, a profile of his family situation would show how his older brother—also a gang member and drug user—paved the way for Juan's delinquent behavior. This type of profiling would also include the contextual influences on Juan's development. For example, Juan's parents consider that a boy of his age should behave responsibly, with minimal or no monitoring of his activities.

Kazdin advocates combined and multimodal treatments that satisfy the requirement of a broader conceptualization of impairment, made up of both specific problems and "contextual conditions."[4] We also support a multimodal approach to intervention, which draws on multiple techniques and types of treatment and which tailors treatment to individual cases.

Expanding the Scope of Psychological Interventions

As described in Chapter Four, a therapist who takes a contextual perspective views psychotherapy itself as a proximal process, that is, face-to-face interactions at the microsystemic level. However, individual psychotherapeutic modalities provide the most restricted context for interventions. There are now a wide array of modalities that both deepen the scope of intervention (by interrelating levels of the environments in which the youth develops) and broaden the range of intervention (by going beyond the microsystemic level). In this chapter we will explore interventions that focus on the mesosystemic level, the linked social contexts described in Chapter Five.

Recent treatment researchers have developed and tested intervention models based on contextual perspectives, some labeled *ecological*[5] or *ecocultural*,[6] and they have described specific interventions, such as multisystemic treatment,[7] multidimensional family therapy,[8] and multimodal therapy.[9] These interventions have been described in manuals and their effectiveness established through research. However, we believe that a clinician can adopt a contextual perspective without necessarily subscribing to any one type of intervention. What must be emphasized is the role of the youth's social system in bringing about change.[10] As earlier chapters have shown, from a contextual viewpoint intervention is a creative process that addresses each new problematic situation by carefully considering the unique characteristics of the relationships among persons, daily activities that exacerbate or mitigate the problem, contexts within which the problem occurs, and particular features of the time period in which the contexts are situated.

Let us consider Hortensia. Her problems can best be appreciated and addressed if we examine diverse situations within various contexts that make up her past and present life. Her story illustrates the complex ways in which problems and situations interrelate across the microsystemic and mesosystemic contextual levels.

Hortensia is an eleven-year-old Cuban girl who arrived in the United States with her grandmother and nine-year-old brother in the most recent wave of boat people (*balseros*). Hortensia's mother (Grandmother's daughter-in-law) is a woman "in the life"—that is, a prostitute—who uses drugs and who neglected and abused the child before giving custody to her father when she was seven. The father, in turn, put Hortensia in the care of his mother. Hortensia was diagnosed with a seizure disorder as a toddler but was never medicated. It also seems that she never received adequate nutrition or health care. Hortensia, her brother, and her grandmother were taken to Guantánamo Bay when the boat in which they were escaping Cuba was intercepted by the United States Coast Guard. At the base, Hortensia's behavior became extremely erratic and she was diagnosed as psychotic. Because of her condition she was given what was called a medical parole priority. Within six months, Grandmother and children were resettled in a city in the U.S. Southwest. However, they were ill-prepared for their resettlement, speaking no English and having very little knowledge of life in this country. Although only fifty years old and formerly very resourceful in providing for her family in Cuba, Grandmother has difficulty negotiating the U.S. health delivery system, using public transportation, finding employment, or getting special education services for the children.

Hortensia's recent behavior problems consist of inappropriate sexualized behavior, nightmares, suicidal threats, destruction of personal belongings, crying spells, overeating, and self-endangering behavior. She demands attention and is jealous if Grandmother's attention is directed toward her brother. Placed in a sixth-grade class, Hortensia initially did not receive English-as-a-second-language classes or special education. She claimed that other children made fun of her and that her only friend was her brother. She often resorted to sexualized behavior to attract his attention.

Hortensia's primary resource is a loving grandmother who is socially isolated because of the circumstances of her escape from Cuba. Apart from the refugee resettlement services they have received, this small family has no resources and is fearful of the unfamiliar urban world around it. Although it is urgent that Hortensia receive the help she needs before puberty, she cannot be helped unless the family becomes better adapted to life in a southwestern city.

Interventions might include these: helping Grandmother to become more effective as a parental figure in a new environment, such as changing aspects of how she and the children relate, how the siblings interact, and how Hortensia relates to her teachers; intervening in key relationships in linked contexts (the family and school, the family and social service agencies, and so on); helping Hortensia's younger brother cope with problems he is experiencing at school; assisting Grandmother to negotiate with school authorities to provide the services that Hortensia needs; and assisting to improve the family's economic situation by linking the family to appropriate agencies that will provide English classes as well as occupational training and job skills for Grandmother.

Assessment of Problems in Linked Contexts

In a contextual approach, the assessment of emotional and behavior problems requires tracking, through linked contexts, of family and community resources. The initial task of the mental health or social service provider is to profile the persons, activities, and contexts implicated in the referral. In individually focused therapies the attempt to change behavior is usually restricted to one or more microsystemic contexts, such as school or family. At the mesosystemic level, the contextual therapist will first attempt to profile the problem in as many activity settings and contexts as possible, using diverse sources: interviews with parents, siblings, extended family members, teachers, and probation officers; review of school records, court documents, educational and psychological assessments, and so on. This is a type of fieldwork like that carried out by anthropologists in ethnographic studies, where data on a particular group of persons and on specific topics, situations, and locales are systematically collected. Each of the profiles—such as an exploration of the family setting that includes the structure and organization of the household and family dynamics and relationships—offers the opportunity to explore links between family as context and other contexts. Resources or assets as well as disabilities or deficits must be assessed.

One study has shown that an increase in a youth's assets in different contexts is associated with a decrease in high-risk behaviors.[11] This study suggests that there is an inverse relationship between assets—such as a warm, concerned family—and risk indicators—such as learning problems. Youths with four risk indicators in the major contexts (family, school, youth activities, and religious or spiritual involvement) generally have no assets, but those who have at least one major asset in one context (for example, doing well in school) will average only three risk indicators, and so on. Although this study was not contextual, it has implications for assessment and intervention. Which assets or risk behaviors should be weighted most heavily when determining the direction of treatment will depend on the profile that the therapist constructs.

Accounting for Differing Perspectives

We can illustrate the importance of a process of assessment that focuses on linked contexts by referring again to Hortensia's family situation. Hortensia's nine-year-old brother, Jaime, offers an example of how a contextual approach to assessment may be particularly important when people in different contexts perceive the situation and the individual in very different ways.

Grandmother perceives Jaime as a loving, charming, ideal "little boy" who is destined to become a ladies' man. When he attended family therapy during a period when his sister was hospitalized, hospital staff perceived Jaime as an exuberant "little clown" who desperately wanted the attention of adults, espe-cially males. At school, his teachers perceive him as a sneaky, rambunctious, hyperactive boy who acts up when adults are not present and later "plays up" to his teachers. When Grandmother filled out a child behavior checklist, no significant problems with attention and impulsiveness were noted. In contrast, his teacher noted significant problems with attention, hyperactivity, and im-pulsiveness. A computerized vigilance test actually showed Jaime to have prob-lems with inattention and hyperactivity. (As we noted earlier, such tests may overestimate problems of Latino youths in this area because standards have been established in tests of non-Latino youth.) In Jaime's case, dealing with his exuberant behavior became a problem because of the varied perspectives on how disruptive or serious it was.

Interviews with Grandmother, sister Hortensia, and Jaime himself show his intense desire to be esteemed and accepted by father figures, confirming the views of the health care providers and suggesting particular avenues of intervention. The therapist learns that Jaime's uncle in Cuba is a martial arts instructor and that Jaime idolizes this uncle and speaks often about his desire to learn martial arts. Training in the martial arts as an additional intervention is suggested and arrangements made for Jaime to earn a scholarship at a local martial arts studio, the scholarship contingent on Jaime maintaining a C aver-age in school and behaving well in the classroom. (The studio owner is a very fatherly man who offers scholarships to disadvantaged youth.) The resulting training provides a paternal surrogate figure for Jaime as well as the opportu-nity for healthy peer relationships and intense—but supervised—activity.

Assessing Family Resources

Jeanne Brooks Gunn's list of family resources include these: in-come, time, human capital, and psychological capital.[12] For exam-ple, in linking family and school one might assess the human capital represented by the parents' education, which heavily in-fluences the outcomes of child development, both in terms of sup-port for education and in association with parental employment and income. As we noted in the last chapter, better-educated Latino parents generally have fewer problems relating both to in-dividual teachers and to the school as a system serving their chil-dren's needs. Moreover, these parents organize their households and their time to facilitate their children's schoolwork and learning. They also have the time and money to provide educational tools (computers, books) and enriching experiences. These resources are culturally patterned in important ways. Many low-income Latino parents who lack education beyond grade school hold teachers in such high regard as to find it difficult to approach them, let alone disagree over educational policies that affect their children. Often, poor immigrant parents assume that community agencies, such as the school, will take responsibility for their children's education or antisocial behavior without expecting or requiring the parents' participation. This assumption is probably associated with the traditional emphasis in Latin American countries on social hierarchies and with the rather rigid boundaries between social classes that empower community agents. These may be the sources of feelings of social disempowerment of parents in extrafamilial contexts.

Assessing Feelings of Difference and Isolation

We believe that it is essential to assess the degree to which Latino youths and their family members—immigrants in particular—perceive themselves to be an integral part of the social environments in which they live. The extent to which this may be a problem depends on a number of factors: if there is a critical mass of Latinos living in the neighborhood, if neighbors are immigrants or U.S.-born, if the Latinos in the neighborhood are culturally homogeneous, and if English is spoken with sufficient fluency to allow interaction with non-Latino neighbors and community institutions.

A Tale of Two Latino Boys

Gerardo and Ricardo were second-generation Mexican Americans born in the same city. Gerardo grew up in a neighborhood composed largely of Mexican immigrants, whereas Ricardo's neighborhood was largely European American. By the time they got to high school, Ricardo was known as Richard, whereas Gerardo kept his Spanish name. Richard associated with either European Americans or other Latinos who were highly identified with European Americans. Gerardo and his friends saw Richard as a *vendido* (a sellout). For Richard's part, despite his efforts to assimilate into mainstream American culture, he had a sense of never having been fully accepted by his European American peers and yet of being alienated from other Mexican Americans. In contrast, Gerardo was well accepted by both sets of peers and did not suffer ethnic identity conflicts.

Because it is important to assess assets and vulnerabilities, the cases of Richard and Gerardo are instructive. At this particular point in their development, Richard may be more susceptible to negative peer influences because of his desire to be accepted or because of negative emotional states such as depression and anger.

The Latino Immigrant Youth in the United States

It is not uncommon to hear Latino immigrant youths complain that they feels rejected by other Latinos who are more highly acculturated. For example, Paco was a member of a group of young adolescents of Mexican origin who met for group psychotherapy. All of the youths except Paco had been born in the United States or lived in the Southwest since the age of four or thereabouts. In contrast, Paco had only been a resident for the past three years and had become fluent in English only during the preceding six months. When he entered the group room, he would always sit in the corner, often with his face averted from the circle of members. The group facilitator, a young woman who identified herself as a Chicana, addressed him in Spanish from time to time to attempt to ensure his comfort if he felt inhibited in using English, but he remained silent through three sessions. At the fourth session, the facilitator noticed that Paco had piled up the bean bags (which were the group's choice for seating) and was sitting high above the other group members. At an appropriate moment, the facilitator jokingly said that Paco was undoubtedly "above" the other group members. He then began to smile as the stack of bean bags became very wobbly. When he finally straightened out his seating and descended to the level of the other youths, he began to disclose his feelings. He said that he felt put down and angry as a Mexican in the United States and that he wanted to return to Mexico. When he felt angry at being made to feel bad about his Mexican origin, he got a huge lump in his throat. Although he usually contained his anger, he disclosed that he had gotten into fights with *Chicanos* because he was a *Mexicano*. He felt different from them, in part because they taunted him about his accent and style of dress. He said, *"Chicanos no son Mexicanos porque son mas Americanos que Mexicanos."*

("Chicanos are not the real thing because they are more American than Mexican.")

When Latino Youths Are Isolated Among Other Latinos

Given the variation in Latino cultures and migration to different parts of the United States, it is not unusual for a Puerto Rican youth, for example, to find himself in a singular position among Mexican American youths in the Southwest or among Mexican immigrant youths in a Texas border town. When Pedro's mother got a job in a southwestern city, Pedro was moved from a school in Connecticut where 70 percent of his classmates were Puerto Rican, and almost all of them spoke Spanish, to a school where only a small number of Mexican-origin youths spoke Spanish with a very different accent and some differences in vocabulary. Pedro's teachers put him under much greater pressure to learn English and he did so to gain acceptance by peers. Perhaps the greatest feeling of difference was the way in which friends related to one another. The Puerto Rican youths that Pedro had known in the Eastern city were accustomed to friends moving between the island and different cities on the mainland United States. They were more open to accepting Puerto Rican newcomers, and they put up fewer boundaries to friendship. Pedro's Puerto Rican friends focused more on Latin Caribbean music and entertainment (salsas and boleros), whereas the Mexican American youths were more focused on Tejano music and popular U.S. music types.

Ease of Communication

Language, and the perception of being an outsider, plays a large part in making Spanish-speaking immigrants feel unwanted or even spurned by those whom they expect will help to raise their children as well as by North Americans in general. One Mexican mother, a five-year U.S. resident, was very focused on learning English. She explained, "They make us feel like *cucarachas* (cockroaches); they would step on us if we let them." She recalled having difficult experiences even with shopgirls who refused to speak Spanish with her although they were clearly Latinas who understood the language. She felt that her ability to be successful in this often-hostile environment depended on acquiring fluency in speaking and reading English. Latinos also often feel like outsiders when they do not become fluent in English despite long residence in the United States because they live in isolated communities (like northern New Mexico) or towns on the border between Mexico and the United States.

Strategies for Intervening Within Linked Contexts

Ecological approaches to interventions target strategies that are directed toward changing activity settings in the environment, rather than in the individual. The ecologically minded therapist might target an environmental factor that has the potential of working quickly and offers the greatest beneficial change in environmental fit. Our formulation of a contextual approach includes targeting strategies that focus on the interaction between a developing youth and social contexts that link his or her daily activities. An exploration of Rogelio's family situation illustrates the importance of linking family and school situations and targeting those factors that have good potential for change.

Rogelio is a ten-year-old Guatemalan boy who was failing in school. His teacher complained that he was often restless, seeking attention from her to explain the assignments. When she asked why he did not get help at home he got upset and refused to answer her.

When first seen, Rogelio's family was living in a homeless shelter, a situation that greatly compromised the family's ability to function well in various life activities. The children complained that they were not able to do their homework, bring friends home, or relax during their free time. The parents responded to their children's complaints with increasing impatience because the complaints signified a lack of "respect" to which all parents are entitled. This sense of "shame" was exacerbated by the frequent presence of the nuns who ran the shelter and sometimes entered into these discussions. Rogelio's father often complained, "I feel like a child in my own family."

It seemed that any attempt to change Rogelio's school performance—given his parents' inability to provide a suitable home environment for their children—would likely fail. In this situation, the linking of contexts in assessing Rogelio's problems led to the cornerstone of a series of interventions on Rogelio's and his family's behalf. His father was helped to acquire a loan to purchase a small plot and a mobile home that provided adequate housing for the family.

Among the newer innovative interventions based on the notions of social ecology, there are several whose effectiveness has been demonstrated by research into outcomes. However, effectiveness for Latino youth—with the notable exception of the treatment research with Cubans (and other Latinos in the Miami area) by José Szapocznik and his colleagues in Florida[13]—has not been explored to any extent. In order to familiarize the reader with contextual approaches, we will briefly describe a few selected programs and apply them to the problems described in Chapter Five. Although these are ecologically oriented interventions and include multiple contexts, they rarely take culture into account in the systematic way we described earlier. In comparison, therapists with a social constructionist perspective view culture (as described in Chapter Four) as situated in the interactions between individuals and particular activity settings and contexts. Our descriptions of the cases that follow are intended to suggest ways in which culture can be integrated into interventions that aim to bring about changes in the linked social contexts that make up a youth's everyday environment.

Family-Based Ecological Interventions

Two different approaches to interventions focused on families in context have become popular since the 1970s. The first, the Family Resource Movement, includes family resource and support programs that emerged out of the 1960s antipoverty campaign and were later influenced by Bronfenbrenner's ecological theory of human development.[14] These programs focus on establishing a social service network of agencies that share in planning and delivering comprehensive services for families and children. An important thrust is that of family support guided by a set of principles that include inspiring parental confidence, responding to family cultural preferences, assisting in problems of living, providing information that parents seek, empowering relationships between families and community agencies or other institutions, and facilitating voluntary parent participation.[15] The Family Resource Movement has been credited with changing social service delivery's emphasis from crisis care to promotion of health and well-being for children and families.

A development within the Family Resource Movement is *home-based therapy,* which, as its name implies, advocates using the home setting as a therapeutic site.[16] The basic idea is that intervening in the home accommodates the needs of lower-income, working, and single parents, as well as of other families who have difficulty getting to an office or clinic. A central principle is that parents should be supported so that they can better fulfill their child-rearing responsibilities. There are a number of advantages to intervening in the home setting: the task of engagement is made easier, access to the family system is enhanced, and new patterns of behavior can be directly introduced and implemented in the family environment. From the perspective of the contextual approach we have described, therapists who intervene in the home can acquire more extensive and detailed knowledge of the family's lifestyle and can better develop ways to be culturally responsive.

Structural Ecosystemic Interventions

The second approach to intervention in linked contexts has arisen through the widespread popularity of family therapy, which most recently has included new approaches such as narrative family therapy,[17] multidimensional family therapy,[18] and *ecosystemic* therapy.[19] Beginning two decades ago with structural and strategic models of family therapy[20] and enhanced by cultural adaptations based on a study of values in the Cuban community, the Spanish Family Guidance Center in Miami developed what its members now view as a contextual approach to prevention and treatment at the mesosystemic and exosystemic levels. They have developed three programs, which they label *structural ecosystemic:* Shenandoah in Action, a school-based program; Little Havana Parent Leadership Program, a community-based program; and the Human Ecology Treatment Program, a comparative study of the effectiveness of an ecologically based treatment program versus a treatment-as-usual approach for adolescent substance users. The core of the Miami group's approach is a focus on repetitive patterns of interaction within and between systems, and the notion that some of these patterns will lead to problem behaviors. For example, the Shenandoah in Action program focuses on correcting maladaptive interactions at micro-, meso-, and exosystemic levels by redirecting youths and other participants "out of conflictive and or nonsupportive interactions into a supportive network of interactional processes."[21] The

Human Ecology Treatment Program addresses goals such as developing a working alliance between parents and schools, helping parents acquire information on the peer activities engaged in by their children, teaching parents how to supervise their children's peer relationships, and attempting to change the peer relationships of drug-abusing youth. The Miami researchers are particularly aware of the problem of cultural conflict as a mediator in the relationship between Latino youths, who are acculturating to North American youth culture, and their parents, who are attempting to maintain some or all of the traditions they learned as children.

Multisystemic Therapy

Multisystemic therapy (MST) is a recent innovative intervention that targets serious antisocial behavior in youths in different populations.[22] It is clearly ecological in approach, but it is based on family systems concepts of behavior and behavior change that begin with a youth's behavior problems and reflect dysfunctional family patterns.[23] Variations on multisystemic therapy have been developed, some with the addition of family preservation, but the main thrust is to carry out intensive interventions at the sites (family, peer, school, and neighborhood contexts) of the youth's activities. Because this type of intervention has been demonstrated to reduce incarceration among frequently violent and chronic criminal offenders by decreasing these youths' aggression with peers, it is clearly cost-effective.[24] Other significant outcomes have been increased warmth and cohesion in the family and decreased youth aggression with peers.

A manual for MST describes the intervention as based on family systems notions of behavior and behavior change but expanded beyond this approach to work with individuals in related contexts; it is also described as "nested" or "embedded" in social systems beyond but connected with the family.

First, strengths and weaknesses of the youths, as well as their transactions within social systems beyond the family, are assessed in family sessions. Problems identified in the family are targeted for change and relevant systems outside the family are assessed for strengths and resources that may help to bring about change. Up to this point the intervention is similar to the multidimensional family therapies cited earlier.[25] However, MST dictates that the duration of treatment should be at least sixty hours of direct contact, on average, over a four-month period—somewhat more than the family and other visits recommended by interventions that focus more on the family. Sessions are held in the home, the school, or other community settings on a flexible schedule, ranging from one session a week to every day, and are available on a twenty-four-hour basis, with preferred times between 8 A.M. and 10 P.M. Families are seen as their schedules permit, which usually means evenings and weekends. A key aspect of the intervention is the process of targeting problems, setting goals for each session, and assigning extensive homework. The work is carried out by treatment teams of three counselors, all of whom have master's degrees in some area of mental health and who receive intensive, short-term, systematic training and ongoing supervision.

The techniques used in MST—particularly that counselors become part of the environmental settings they help to change—facilitate an in-depth understanding of contexts that is unavailable to therapists who work in clinics, which by their nature are very separate from the sites and settings of the daily life of clients. However, Richard Munger points out that mental health professionals are not routinely trained to deal with ecosystems and therefore are not usually successful in implementing interventions that address multiple social contexts.[26] We might note that therapists also are not accustomed to inquiring into the explanations that clients give for their behavior nor interested in the mundane aspects of everyday life that make up the activities, events, and other behavior significant for gaining a perspective on a youth's development.

Alternative and Traditional Healing Practices as Contextual Interventions

A contextual approach raises the question, "Is mental health the domain of mental health providers alone?" Some ecologically oriented therapists refer to a child's environment as a "natural therapy system."[27] That is, most of the time youths and their environments are sufficiently matched when it comes to a youth's attributes and developmental needs. If problems are identified, it is assumed that there is some impasse in their environments or situations. If this perspective is taken, there is no clear-cut division between mental health care services and other types of therapeutic systems.

Latino traditional and folk healing practices were briefly described in Chapter One. The primary traditional healing systems, *Curanderismo, Espiritismo,* and *Santería* (each with many variations), approached healing from a contextual standpoint long before the social ecology or social constructionist approaches to intervention in North American psychology were developed. Traditional healers (Mexican *curanderos,* Puerto Rican *espiritistas,* and Cuban *santeros*) are mainly seen by adults, much less frequently by children and adolescents. Although *curanderos* commonly treat children with digestive disorders or other physical ailments, they more rarely deal with emotional distress except as secondary to somatic problems. Because the definitions and meanings traditional healing systems give to experiences and symptoms of illness differ from those of biomedicine, psychology, and psychiatry, complaints of bodily distress are considered by these disciplines to be substitutes for what they label as psychological distress.

When emotional distress or deviant behavior is the issue, most Latino healers treat children and adolescents through their parent or parents, who usually take responsibility for both the cause of the distress and the cure. (However, responsibility is shared with distress-causing spirits and other extraordinary beings.) In what follows, we describe a case of prolonged bereavement and a psychotic-like episode in a Puerto Rican girl in order to illustrate how an *espiritista* (a spirit medium-healer) would treat these problems. This case illustrates some of the ways in which traditional healers employ a contextual approach and also frequently consider developmental issues in assessment and treatment.

> Normita was fourteen years old and in a special education class when one day at school she suffered an *ataque de llanto* (a sudden but prolonged crying spell) with intermittent screaming. When her teacher could not get her to stop crying, her mother was summoned to school. Normita eventually calmed down after being taken home. The school counselor referred her to emergency community mental health services, and Normita and her mother were accompanied to the community mental health center by the counselor on the following day. However, just before leaving home for the appointment, Normita took three 10-milligram Valium tablets, which she found in the medicine cabinet.

Normita's family history was supplied by her mother. Normita was the sixth of ten siblings, seven of whom were living at home at the time. One of the siblings, a sister who had been eight years older than Normita, had died some six years earlier. The official cause of death was reported as a brain tumor. However, Mother reported that the death seemed mysterious to the children because it occurred suddenly, in the middle of the night, and the customary death rites—such as eight nights of rosaries or a viewing of the body—had not occurred. Normita's father had been a recovering alcoholic and mental health patient for five years before this sister died, and the family had been subsisting on social security disability payments. They could not afford the expenses of the funeral rites. At school, Normita had always had learning problems, and she was often withdrawn and sad.

At her initial clinic visit, Normita told her therapist that shortly after her sister died the girl's spirit had begun to appear each night at Normita's bedside. Normita had a very close relationship with this sister. They had slept in the same bed, and the sister had helped her with her homework and looked after most of her needs. The spirit's appearance did not distress Normita during these six years. However, in recent months the sister's spirit had begun warning Normita to get away from their father because he was "Satan" and would harm her. Normita had not previously told anyone about these experiences because she had not been frightened by them until recently.

Before the sister's death, the father had been physically abusing his wife and the older children. Normita's favorite, the deceased sister, had been a special target of her father's attacks, and Normita appeared to blame him for the girl's death. When the therapist spoke about these events to Normita's mother, she seemed passive and unresponsive to Normita's needs. Even though the father was no longer drinking, he remained emotionally distant, rigid, and authoritarian. Moreover, her mother and siblings considered Normita to be normal despite her school problems, frequent social withdrawal at home, and her recent *ataque*.

In family sessions Normita's therapist and the family members discussed their feelings about the older sister's death, opening what had formerly been a forbidden topic. The therapist arranged a visit to the grave and sought to convince Normita that her sister's death was a natural event and that she had nothing to fear from her father. The sister's spirit was labeled a psychological phenomenon, an illusion that could be dealt with symbolically because it was a projection of Normita's fear and hostility toward her father.

However, when Normita did not seem to respond to therapy and remained withdrawn and highly anxious, her mother took her to a traditional healer, an *espiritista,* who worked at a local Spiritist center. The healer's intervention strategy differed considerably from that of the therapist.

The spirit mediums at the center to which Normita went considered the spirit to be real. In their view, the sister was distressed and her spirit's fluids had entered Normita's body, resulting in her feelings of hostility and fear. (This is a notion about contagion of the sister's feelings and also of the illness from which the sister died.) They first "took off" (*despojos*) the sister's spirit by calling the spirit to the table where they were working and then sweeping Normita's body with their arms in an attempt to relieve Normita of the spirit's impress on her body. However, when this healing technique was not effective, they decided that the spirit had come to help Normita as a spiritual guide. Their explanation was that they understood Normita's feelings of abandonment and anger around the loss of her sister and recognized that her mother did not provide the sense of caring and security that Normita needed—especially now that she was on the threshold of puberty with its attendant doubts and confusion. They concluded that the spirit of the mother who had given birth to Normita in a previous life had come again to support and nurture her. They blamed the father for the chaos the family had suffered in the past and felt he was reaping the evil he had sown over many past lives by being rejected by his children and particularly by Normita's hostility and accusations.

In essence, the healers were trying to help Normita let go of her intense negative emotional involvement with her father by indirectly suggesting that he needed to be ignored or barely tolerated rather than feared. They emphasized the need for the girl to have someone in whom to confide; someone to tell that she felt as if she had been buried in a cement box and could not escape her isolation. And they said that she was in development to be a spirit medium, assisted by the maternal spirit of her dead sister as her principal spirit guide. This meant that she was being invited to attend the inner circle of the mediums at that center as a novitiate. By doing this, she would acquire mother surrogates among the mediums practicing at that center, who would be her spiritual mentors, in addition to the spirit-guide mother that she already had.

These healers appeared to be aware of the need to change or readjust interactions in linked contexts (that is, the family, the healing center, and the spirit world). The suggestion that Normita become a medium was unusual for one so young but it added a social setting and network that were missing in her family life. It is worth noting that some mental health practitioners might have diagnosed her as having a psychotic disorder, which would have meant hospitalization and a psychiatric patient label. The healers combined what we would view as ecological and social constructionist intervention strategies: they suggested, through spirit intervention, a new social context for Normita, in which what might have been seen as a weakness (her visions of the dead sister) would be redefined as a strength (her potential ability to develop as a spirit medium).

Our Approach to Linked Contexts: A Case Example

As we described in Chapter Two, our approach to formulating and carrying out interventions with Latino youth combines ecological and social constructionist perspectives. If we take the earlier-mentioned Juan as an example, an ecological perspective suggests a set of interventions engaging the linked contexts of some of his problems—family and school. Juan also has problems when it comes to his choice of friends, who encourage him to engage in antisocial behavior. In the following case description, we only consider this context of his problem behavior in relation to his school problems. In describing the direction that intervention might take in Juan's case, we consider culture as an integral part of the contexts toward which the interventions are targeted. We strongly suggest that recommendations for changing interactions among the client and the people in his or her environments not be imposed on either the client or the situations. Nor should the therapist prescribe how to change these contexts (that is, the family and school environments) based on some implicit or explicit notion (norm) about what constitutes appropriate behavior for a youth of Juan's age and gender. Instead, at the mesosystemic level, the therapist should allow the planning for the direction of change in activities, persons, or situations to emerge out of a process of eliciting the views on Juan's problem behavior of his parents, his teacher, and his counselor, and Juan himself. In addition, the therapist needs to consider the quality of the interactions between Juan and his parents in various settings of daily activity (for example, the amount of monitoring they give his activities), the arrangement of activity settings in each context (for example, the time spent assisting Juan with his homework and the space set aside for doing homework), and the relationship between contexts (for example, the participation of each parent in teacher conferences).[28] The therapist would then negotiate change in the ways in which Juan, his parents, and his teachers interact, always focusing on their ideas about what types of change would be effective.

We will describe this process in more detail after providing more facts about Juan.

> When first referred for help Juan was thirteen years old. He reported that he had been smoking pot for about a year, had tried "meths" (methamphetamine), and had also started smoking cigarettes a year ago. He had almost continuous difficulty with school since the early grades—was restless in class, impulsive, and talked out of turn. Because of many absences, he had been suspended three times over the past year. Both at home and at school, Juan appeared easily irritated and resentful, often used obscene language, and was argumentative and prone to temper tantrums. Among other phobic reactions, Juan reported being afraid of school—of speaking, writing, or reading in front of others.

When systematically explored as a profile of problems, it seems clear that in addition to conduct problems and phobias Juan has problems of impulsivity and hyperactivity that have affected his performance throughout his school career. Given the circumstances of the family moving from Mexico to Los Angeles and then to the Southwest, Juan's problems in the classroom appear never to have been remediated, perhaps overlooked by a focus on his conduct problems. His teachers believe that because of his failures at school he associates with youths who are members of a gang, youths who espouse the attitude that school is meaningless and that real life means being autonomous on the streets. Juan reports that he drinks and does drugs when he feels bad. He has seriously overdosed on alcohol on at least two occasions. He blacked out at those times and was hospitalized in a coma on the last occasion.

Assessment and Intervention as a Single Process

If we were to attempt to change Juan's problematic experiences both at school and in the family, in order to improve his chances of staying in school as well as lessen conflict between him and his parents, it would take several types of interventions, involving his parents and siblings, his teachers, the school counselor, and other school personnel as indicated by the school. Intervening in all of these contexts is the goal of ecologically oriented family therapies. However, in addition to this approach, if we took a contextual perspective we would conduct a process of assessment using a method of nonjudgmental, open-ended inquiry. We might first attempt to enter Juan's world, explore with him his personal characteristics (temperament, for example), his strengths and resources (such as his close relationship with his family and loyalty to them). In addition, we might assess Juan's views on the activities and situations that were reported as problematic. (A full description of this process, at the level of the individual client, was given in Chapter Four.)

When dealing with linked contexts, we would then seek to understand Juan's parents' and siblings' worlds, as well as the situation of the family at the intersection of these worlds. We might then try to engage Juan's parents in a dialogue that would yield an in-depth understanding of attitudes, values, and interpretations around educational experience in general and, more specifically, their views on the school system and its characteristics in the United States that have been influential in their notions about schooling for their children. In entering into this dialogue, we might covertly raise a number of questions (that is, raise them in our own minds). Do Juan's parents feel that a high school education is essential for their son? How responsible do they feel for Juan's behavior in school? Do they blame the school personnel for not informing them about his problems in a timely manner or for dealing with him through punitive measures such as suspension? Do they feel intimidated about going to school and discussing Juan's problems? Are they afraid that their command of English is inadequate to the task? Are they reluctant to seek help from school personnel because they feel socially inferior to Juan's teachers and counselor? Do they think that Juan has the ability to do better work at school? Do they think that Juan should be able to control his impulsivity and be more successful in school?

These and many other questions might suggest themselves; however, they should remain unverbalized to avoid biasing the parents' responses. We suggest that the therapist's role in assessing persons, activities, and contexts is to act as a humble inquirer who allows answers to these kinds of questions to emerge from the inquiry. Initially we might ask some very broad questions, such as: Could you tell me about your experiences with Juan in relation to school (or at home)? As the interview proceeds and the interviewee's perspectives have been amply expressed, more detailed questions can be introduced where clarifications of views or attitudes are needed, or when deepening a particular subject seems necessary to formulating the type and direction of the interventions.

Once we understand the perspectives of both Juan and his parents, a next step might be to have Juan and his parents discuss their views with one another in order to explore possible common ground (defined as an area in which their views coincide). For example, do his parents understand why school experiences are difficult for Juan in the way that Juan understands this problem? How do school experiences relate to his behavior and attitudes toward school, to his interactions with family members and peers, or to activities in other life arenas? The assumption we make in suggesting this approach is that common ground will emerge with sufficient exploration of activities, contexts, and perspectives and explanations of participants. Rather than acting as a negotiator between different views and interpretations, the therapist should act as an explorer looking for descriptions of aspects of clients' lifescapes that eventually might yield mutually held views.

We suggest that the process of inquiry itself is therapeutic and can produce change in persons-in-activities-in-context. For example, as the dialogues of the participants interviewed yield pieces of lifescapes that are similar to one another, it demonstrates that the youth and the parents share similar views. Their discussions lead to an agreement that can reduce areas of interpersonal conflict. Juan's case is important as it pertains to the presence of conflict not just between himself and his parents but also between his parents themselves. Reaching common understandings with their son may offer them a way to relate differently to each other.

The third step in the process of assessment in linked contexts is to conduct a dialogue with Juan's teacher or other involved school personnel in a manner regulated by the school. We conduct an inquiry into the teacher's and counselor's views of Juan, especially in relation to his activities in the school setting. Once these views are elicited without imposing ideas or posing leading questions, we might then set up a meeting or meetings between Juan, his parents, his teacher or teachers, and other school personnel—a fourth step. Doing this requires Juan's consent and, ideally, his presence, in focusing on the main area of concern: his failure at school. Central to this process is the need to profile Juan's strengths and assets in order to offset the negative views of him as a person as well as to suggest changes in his activities and activity settings. For example, Juan has demonstrated some talent for the guitar but has had little training or opportunity to see if he could gain satisfaction from or excel in this activity. Although he has difficulties with basic scholarship, success as a school musician could motivate him to stay in school and accept other types of interventions, such as private tutoring in mathematics. Again, common ground in the views of all the participants in Juan's world (now including the school) must be sought to chart the direction and type of interventions in activity settings in order to deal with his problem behavior at home and school.

Although his parents and teachers are all concerned about Juan's substance use and gang membership, they might agree to refer Juan and his parents to a local Latino counseling center in order not to overwhelm or shame Juan by discussing these topics among so many authority figures. At a separate site for specific intervention in these problems, the therapist, parents, and Juan might hold a further dialogue, again seeking some common ground that might lead to group therapy for substance abuse, to a community-based program for gang prevention, or to family therapy at the Latino counseling center. A case manager might be enlisted to assist Juan and his family to enroll in these programs and coordinate the array of services they are receiving.

Intervention into Juan's Problems

The next step is to formulate interventions based on the multi-dimensional process of inquiry described. (This process ideally continues even as the interventions take place.) It is important to mention again that tapping into the participants' local worlds includes their culture: that is, the particular activities that structure their lives and the meanings associated with these activities (from an anthropological perspective we might term them *cultural practices.*)

A therapist might first hold a number of sessions with Juan's parents, siblings, and Juan himself (in various combinations) in part to support the parents in the activity of taking their views of his problems to his teachers and counselors but also to engage Juan's siblings in the hope that they will encourage him to participate in the interventions. The parents might be helped to assert themselves at school and ask that Juan be assessed to understand better his strengths and weaknesses. Given the lack of fluency in English and perceptions of social distance between the parents and school personnel, a new system of interaction would need to be introduced into the situation. For example, we might translate (perhaps with the help of a more fluent older sibling) after having carefully established a relationship of *confianza* (trust) with the parents.

Although his parents' concern for him is one of Juan's major assets, in his case we must take into consideration the fact that his parents are in conflict with each other a good part of the time. The conflict stems from their personal relationship rather than from family roles and responsibilities. One might hypothesize that this influences their capacity to control the activities of their sons outside of the home, and this might be changed by working on the parents' relationship. Unfortunately, although their relationship is strong when it comes to cooperating to help their children, it is overwhelmed by the father's resentment of the mother's claim to more personal freedom than he can accept in his marriage. She frequently socializes with friends and claims the freedom to dispose of her own income as she deems necessary, an income that she acquires through well-remunerated work in an electronics factory. This issue involves culture conflict in the sense that marital roles in many immigrant families are affected by situations germane to the availability of employment for women and a change in their attitudes about their status in marriage.[29]

Engaging Fathers

Juan's father's concern about his status brings to the fore one of the more difficult aspects of dealing with Latino families in linked contexts: engaging and retaining fathers in interventions involving school and family.[30] Stereotypes of Latino family patterns and roles (across diverse Latino cultures) hold that the father is the dominant parent and undisputed master in the family. Moreover, he is reported in some studies as emotionally distant from his children and thus marginal to child rearing because he delegates authority to his wife, who deals with the children almost exclusively.[31] Father is said to be concerned about his macho image (that is, his value as a strong and virile man who does not concern himself with daily details and the behavior of young children). As a result of this stereotypical image of the father's role in the family, therapists and others usually select the mother as the target of school and community programs, including parent education and support programs.[32] An alternative view of the father's role in Latino families is that parents have a more egalitarian relationship in family decision making and parenting. A few studies have found fathers in Mexico to be more nurturing and playful with younger children than mothers.[33]

In designing and piloting a parent education project with low-income fathers of Mexican origin, researchers reported six lessons they learned about engaging fathers: project staff must have a firm commitment to working with men; spouses are interdependent participants, with the wife being an informal gatekeeper of the husband's involvement; problem-solving styles should be tailored to men's ways of relating to others; the implications for the women of involving their husbands and other men (strangers) must be considered and dealt with; the roles assigned to men should be unique and respect their self-definitions; and issues of high interest to men—such as conditions that affect their job or their income or access to health care or other services for their families—should be included in the program. These ideas are very relevant to family-based, multidimensional therapies, where it is crucial to consider how to engage both parents. Recognizing a father's leadership role in the family as a critical element can in many cases be a convincing way to engage him in family therapy, if his wife cooperates fully. Returning to the case of Juan, we observed that Father felt his leadership role threatened both by his wife's attempts at independence and by the disturbing behavior of his sons, who no longer obeyed him without question. For treatment to be successful, Father had to be convinced that he was essential to any plan to intervene in Juan's problem behavior.

Apart from changing activities directly related to conflict in the family or to school problems, we must carefully consider Juan's report that activities with his delinquent peers bring satisfaction; they may be among the few things that "make him feel good." Recent stays in juvenile detention have scared him, and he made a point during one family therapy session to say that one of his best friends was in an adult jail for at least five years. He felt sad and afraid for him. Although it appears that stealing has served as a symbolic act of defiance for Juan, an act of solidarity with his *homeboys*—that is, his fellow gang members—and a means to buy drugs on occasion, one point of common ground among his parents and teachers has been the observation that work, and therefore a salary, may meet his needs for autonomy and self-determination. His parents and teachers expressed the view that he had the social skills to take on a job that did not require advanced special training, such as working in a fast food restaurant or supermarket warehouse. Moreover, as mentioned earlier, Juan had fathered a child. Providing for this child could be an additional motivator for Juan to enter a job mentorship program through his school. Time in this program could be counted toward the hours and credits he needs to complete high school. In Juan's parents' view, being financially responsible for a child is a key characteristic of the "good and mature man," and his father has amply modeled this behavior.

Conclusion

In our formulation of a contextual approach to interventions, the process of inquiry used to arrive at the kinds of interventions to employ in particular activity settings should take center stage. In this chapter and in Chapter Four, we advanced this idea primarily because it makes cultures and their variations accessible to the therapist. It also aligns the therapist with the local worlds, experiences, and understandings of a youth with problems related to poor fit with his environment and with persons in contexts and activity settings significant to his development.

In this chapter, we have explored and described a series of suggested steps in a process by which interventions are chosen or developed. In Chapter Seven, we will expand our ideas regarding the arena for interventions by exploring the neighborhood and community as contexts for activities and activity settings. We will also examine dimensions of the lifescapes of youths and their family members, including religious activities and spirituality, to which we have so far given relatively little attention.

Notes

1. A. E. Kazdin, "Combined and Multimodal Treatments in Child and Adolescent Psychotherapy: Issues, Challenges, and Research Directions," *Clinical Psychology: Science and Practice, 3*(1) (1996): 69–100.
2. R. L. Munger, "Ecological Trajectories in Child Mental Health," in *Innovative Approaches for Difficult-to-Treat Populations,* ed. S. W. Henggeler and A. B. Santos (Washington, D.C.: American Psychiatric Press, 1997), 3–25.
3. Kazdin, "Combined and Multimodal Treatments."
4. Kazdin, "Combined and Multimodal Treatments," p. 73.
5. Munger, "Ecological Trajectories."
6. T. S. Weisner, "The Ecocultural Project of Human Development," *Ethos, 25*(2) (June 1997): 177–190.
7. S. W. Henggeler and C. M. Borduin, *Family Therapy and Beyond: A Multisystemic Approach to Treating the Behavior Problems of Children and Adolescents* (Pacific Grove, Calif.: Brooks/Cole, 1990).
8. National Institute on Drug Abuse, *Clinical Report and Administrators Guide to Drug Abuse Treatment Models,* NIDA monograph (Washington, D.C.: U.S. Government Printing Office, 1995); J. L. Lebo and A. S. Gurman, "Research Assessing Couple and Family Therapy," *Annual Reviews of Psychology, 46* (1995): 27–57; H. A. Liddle, "Conceptual and Clinical Dimensions of a Multidimensional, Multisystems Engagement Strategy in Family-Based Adolescent Treatment," *Psychotherapy, 32* (1995): 39–58; H. A. Liddle, "Family-Based Treatment for Adolescent Behavior Problems: Overview of Contemporary Developments and Introduction to the Special Section," *Journal of Family Psychology, 10*(1) (Mar. 1996): 3–11.

9. Kazdin, "Combined and Multimodal Treatments."

10. Munger, "Ecological Trajectories."

11. P. Benson, *The Troubled Journey: A Portrait of 6th to 12th Grade Youth* (Minneapolis, Minn.: Lutheran Brotherhood, 1990).

12. J. Brooks Gunn, "Children in Families and Communities: Risk and Intervention in the Bronfenbrenner Tradition," in *Examining Lives in Context: Perspectives on the Ecology of Human Development,* ed. P. Moen, G. H. Elder Jr., and K. Lüscher (Washington, D.C.: American Psychological Association, 1995), chap. 14.

13. J. Szapocznik and others, "The Evolution of Structural Ecosystemic Theory for Working with Latino Families," *Psychological Interventions and Research with Latino Populations,* ed. J. G. Garcia and M. C. Zea (Needham Heights, Mass.: Allyn & Bacon, 1997), 166–190.

14. B. Weissbourd, "The Evolution of the Family Resource Movement," in *Putting Families First: America's Family Support Movement and the Challenge of Change,* ed. S. L. Kagan and B. Weissbourd (San Francisco: Jossey-Bass, 1994).

15. B. T. Bowman, "Home and School: The Unresolved Relationship," in *Putting Families First: America's Family Support Movement and the Challenge of Change,* ed. S. L. Kagan and B. Weissbourd (San Francisco: Jossey-Bass, 1994).

16. L. J. Wood, "Home-Based Family Therapy," *Social Work, 33*(3) (May-June 1988): 211–214.

17. S. de Shazer, *Words Were Originally Magic* (New York: Norton, 1994).

18. H. A. Liddle, "Family-Based Treatment for Adolescent Problem Behaviors: Overviews of Contemporary Developments and Introduction to the Special Section," *Journal of Family Psychology, 10*(1) (Mar. 1996): 3–11.

19. Szapocznik and others, "The Evolution of Structural Ecosystemic Theory."

20. S. Minuchin, *Families and Family Therapy* (Cambridge, Mass.: Harvard University Press, 1974); C. Madanes, *Strategic Family Therapy* (San Francisco: Jossey-Bass, 1981).

21. Szapocznik and others, "The Evolution of Structural Ecosystemic Theory."

22. Henggeler and Borduin, *Family Therapy and Beyond;* S. W. Henggeler, G. B. Melton, and L. A. Smith, "Family Preservation Using Multisystemic Therapy: An Effective Alternative to Incarcerating Serious Juvenile Offenders," *Journal of Consulting and Clinical Psychology, 60*(6) (1992): 953–961.

23. S. G. Pickrel, J. A. Hall, and P. B. Cunningham, "Interventions for Adolescents Who Abuse Substances," in *Innovative Approaches for*

Difficult-to-Treat Populations, ed. S. W. Henggler and A. B. Santos (Washington, D.C.: American Psychiatric Press, 1997).

24. Henggeler, Melton, and Smith, "Family Preservation Using Multisystemic Therapy."
25. Liddle, "Family-Based Treatment for Adolescent Behavior"; Szapocznik and others, "The Evolution of Structural Ecosystemic Theory."
26. Munger, "Ecological Trajectories."
27. Munger, "Ecological Trajectories."
28. Munger, "Ecological Trajectories."
29. C. Falicov, "Mexican Families," in *Ethnicity and Family Therapy,* ed. M. McGoldrick, J. K. Pearce, and J. Giordana (New York: Guilford Press, 1982), 134–163.
30. D. R. Powell, "Including Latino Fathers in Parent Education and Support Programs," in *Understanding Latino Families: Scholarship, Policy and Practice,* ed. R. Zambrana (Thousand Oaks, Calif.: Sage, 1995), chap. 5.
31. P. Bronstein, "Differences in Mother's and Father's Behavior Toward Children: A Cross-Cultural Comparison," *Developmental Psychology, 20*(6) (1984): 995–1003.
32. Powell, "Including Latino Fathers."
33. Bronstein, "Differences in Mother's and Father's Behavior."

Chapter Seven

Intervening in Community Contexts

Staring at a skyscraper reaching into heaven,
When over in the ghetto I'm living in hell.
PLACIDO VASQUEZ JR.

A boy who presents to a mental health agency because he feels depressed, powerless to deal with the domestic violence in the family, ineffective in resisting the pressures to join a gang, and unable to succeed academically at school, may find some help and respite in individual or family therapy sessions. However, making changes that improve his situation and sustaining these changes once therapy ends may require involvement beyond the microsystemic and mesosystemic levels. It then becomes important to conceptualize interventions that include broader contexts and to view the therapist's role as extending into these contexts. We believe that this is especially important for mental health practitioners working with Latino or other ethnic minority youth.

This chapter explores interventions at the *exosystemic level,* which is made up of linkages between two or more institutional settings, only one of which includes the individual. Interventions at the mesosystemic (linked personal contexts) and the exosystemic levels recently have received increasing attention from several ecologically oriented practitioner-researchers mentioned in Chapter Six.[1] In addition, researchers, consultants, and administrators in mental health delivery systems such as Robert Friedman,[2] Kimberly Hoagwood,[3] Judith C. Meyers,[4] and Jerome H. Hanley[5] have emphasized large-scale implementation and institutionalization of flexible, comprehensive, community-oriented, neighborhood-based interventions.

Ecological models that address community contexts have been used to explain some of the widespread problems—such as violence, maltreatment, and substance use—that the youth of today confront. Although these models do not focus on contextual interventions, they have implications for their development. For example, psychologists Dante Cicchetti and Michael Lynch have described an ecological transactional model of community violence and child maltreatment in which they show how the characteristics of the maltreated child and aspects of the microsystem, the exosystem, and the macrosystem interact.[6] Their model focuses on transactions among two types of risk factors for maltreatment: potentiating factors that increase the likelihood of maltreatment and compensatory factors that decrease the likelihood of maltreatment. The discussion of community factors within the exosystem that appear to be associated with violence and maltreatment is particularly intriguing. Among the findings of studies they reviewed were the following:

- Exposure to violence was related to symptoms of distress in children, such as depression and anxiety, but this effect appears to be mediated by the mother's educational level (violence-exposed children with the less-educated mothers suffered more distress).
- Parents who maltreat their children are more likely to be unemployed. The majority of chronically maltreating families are from the lowest socioeconomic levels (although the authors point out that maltreatment is not restricted to families living in poverty).
- Social isolation (lack of social supports and extended family) is also associated with maltreatment. Social isolation may prevent maltreating parents from improving child-rearing practices because they are not exposed to new information through educational institutions, the media, or social networks.
- Parents who are dissatisfied with the social supports in their communities are likely to be dissatisfied with their roles as caregivers and to have poorer interactions with their children.

Based on this information, a contextual practitioner working with a maltreated child or a child at risk for being maltreated might focus on helping the parents find employment; helping the family develop a supportive network in the community (for example, through church, parent-advocacy, or parent-support groups), including renewing extended family ties, providing the family with opportunities for parent training to improve child-rearing practices and parent-child interactions (such as Parents Anonymous); and perhaps even helping the family find housing in a more suitable neighborhood.

Most ecological models of social problems such as abuse and violence do not explain how culture is related to these problems. Consequently, ecologically oriented interventions based on these models do not specify the ways in which they are culturally responsive. The assumption that interventions will be culturally responsive if they are community-oriented and neighborhood-based may be tenable. Nonetheless, if the ways in which these interventions are culturally responsive are not specified then it is difficult to inform practitioners what aspects of intervention need to be considered in order to address the needs and complexities of particular cultural groups.

This chapter explores how contextually oriented interventions at the community level can be culturally responsive to Latino youth. We first describe changes in current mental health practice that either reflect contextual perspectives or are conducive to contextual approaches that extend to the exosystem. Next, we examine statutes and ethical standards as institutionalized cultural practices that guide the conduct of practitioners at the community level. We then consider how clinical practice is influenced by the exosystem.

Changes in Mental Health Practices Underscore Limitations of Individual Therapies

Two recent changes in mental health practices underscore the increasing recognition of the limitations of models of intervention based on individual-focused or family-focused theories.

One change has been the increasing importance given to contextualization of assessment and practice. In Chapter Three, we described how it has recently been recognized that diagnosis alone (a product of symptom configuration and symptom severity) is not sufficient to determine the need for services. Diagnosis combined with level of impairment justifies need for service. As we mentioned previously, this growing phenomenon acknowledges the need to address context in the assessment and treatment of behavioral and emotional problems. For example, one popular instrument that assesses level of impairment is the Child and Adolescent Functional Assessment Scale (CAFAS).[7] The CAFAS rates impairment in children and adolescents across eight scales: role performance at school/work, role performance at home, role performance in the community; behavior toward others, moods/emotions, self-harmful behavior, substance use, and thinking. In addition, it assesses the resources of the youth's caregivers on two other scales: material needs and family/social support. As Kay Hodges, CAFAS developer, indicates, federal guidelines define seriously emotionally disturbed youth as meeting diagnostic criteria (using the most recent version of the *Diagnostic and Statistical Manual*) that specifies "functional impairment . . . in family, school, or community activities."[8]

Another indication that practice is becoming contextualized is the way that assessment of youth has changed over the course of several decades. There was a time when a "complete assessment" of a youth meant a battery of tests, including intellectual, achievement, and personality measures (such as the Thematic Apperception Test or the Children's Apperception Test, the Rorschach Projective Technique, sentence completion, and projective drawings), as well as a quick neuropsychological screen, such as the Bender Visual-Motor Gestalt Test,[9] the Developmental Test of Visual Motor Integration,[10] or the Revised Visual Retention Test.[11] However, in the area of child and adolescent assessment, the move has been toward assessing a child by obtaining data from multiple informants (such as parents and teachers), using behavioral rating scales of the youth in diverse contexts (such as home and school), and observing the youth's behavior in varied contexts at different time periods, in addition to collecting information from the youth (as in an interview or a self-report questionnaire). For example, in assessing whether a child might have an attention-deficit hyperactivity disorder, an evaluator might administer a computerized vigilance test like the Continuous Performance Test to assess the child's ability to attend and concentrate, ask the parents and the child's teachers to complete behavioral rating scales of the child's behavior at home and at school, and observe the child's behavior with different adults (parent, evaluator, teacher) at different times. The child is also likely to be interviewed and given a battery of tests that include measures of cognitive and emotional functioning and achievement as well as neuropsychological screening tests.

The second change in clinical practice is the result of a national movement in mental health care services for youth that was spurred, in part, by Jane Knitzer's seminal book *Unclaimed Children*, which documented the underidentification of children with serious emotional disorders and the inappropriate services these children received.[12] Subsequently, the Child and Adolescent Service System Program (CASSP) of the National Institute of Mental Health (NIMH) helped to direct much-needed attention to children with serious emotional disturbances and their families. In 1986, Beth A. Stroul and Robert M. Friedman published a monograph on community-based systems of care throughout the United States and emphasized the need for organized, multiagency, integrated systems of care.[13]

A concept often linked with the CASSP movement is that of *wraparound*, which refers to the process of supporting children by wrapping—or individualizing—multiple services around them with the help of case managers instead of putting children in institutions.[14] Examples of comprehensive wraparound services are Project Wraparound in Vermont, the Ventura County Planning Model, and Kaleidoscope, Inc. in Chicago.[15] These programs emphasize interagency collaborations and linkages and delineate how the agencies will work together to reduce clients' symptoms and level of impairment. Some of these programs combine the staffs and funds of various agencies and establish formal interagency agreements and interorganizational structures to create integrated programs.

Nevertheless, despite the changes in mental health care delivery since the early 1980s, youths remain underserved. Only about two-thirds of youths in need of mental health services are receiving them, and about 5 percent of these youths may have serious emotional disorders with impairment that precludes age-appropriate functioning.[16] In 1992, Congress authorized the Comprehensive Community Mental Health Services for Children Program and appropriated $60 million for demonstration grants to improve mental health service delivery through "systems of care." This program, which is managed by the Center for Mental Health Services (CMHS), aims "to provide families with services that are both affordable and available when and where they need them."[17] It is guided by the philosophy that families are partners in designing services, focuses on the strengths of children and their families, and respects the race, culture, and ethnicity of youths and their families. CMHS currently manages twenty-two demonstration grants in twenty-nine communities in eighteen states. Its projects, which coordinate systems of care that include mental health, child welfare, education, juvenile justice, and other local public and private agencies, provide a wide array of services that were either underdeveloped or did not exist in the local communities.[18]

To the degree that wraparound community-based services are both effective and economical, managed care organizations and other third-party payers are likely to view them as consistent with their preventative health orientation. Thus, we currently have an economic and health system climate that may actually encourage the development of contextualized mental health treatment. What is lacking is an explication of how contextualized mental health care practices might better take culture into account. Nonetheless, one cannot deny that by taking a look at a youth outside of the office, clinic, or hospital, a practitioner may have to take cultural aspects into account—for example, to address why Alberto is so demanding at home with his mother, who is overprotective and very nurturing, yet anxious and oppositional at school with his non-Latino teacher, who is academically demanding and emotionally aloof.

Statutes and Ethical Standards Are Institutionalized Cultural Practices

In mental health we have statutes and ethical standards that speak to important concerns, such as consent for treatment and release of information. For children, parents' signatures are required for these releases. Many of these statutes and standards are based on the premise that a family is headed by either one or both parents and that any decision about children should have parental consent. However, this premise may be incorrect in cultures in which important caretaking roles are carried out by others. For example, a child may have an extended family in which grandparents or other family members assume roles as the family patriarch or matriarch. These relatives may be routinely consulted by the child's parents for important family decisions. It may be crucial for mental health practitioners to include these persons when the parents have to make important decisions about their children, such as a decision to place a child in a treatment foster home, inpatient unit, or day treatment program, or to obtain consent for family preservation or home-based therapy services. A practitioner should not assume that compliance with a legal requirement such as obtaining the signature of one parent constitutes good practice when treating Latino youths.

In addition, statutes and ethical standards reflect the values and beliefs of a society at a specific period in time. For example, it is unlikely that the concept of privileged communication would had been extended to statutes applying to psychotherapy if the predominant theory in mental health had been behavioral as opposed to psychodynamic. At the time when many such statutes were adopted, psychodynamic approaches emphasized that the unconscious mind could "hide" information from the conscious mind. Thus, it was believed that it was necessary to have a very private and protected special relationship with a therapist in order to uncover the client's unconscious content safely. Unless statutes protected privileged communications and ethical standards guarded confidentiality, it was believed that therapy could not be conducted effectively. Statutes and ethical standards have to be understood within the zeitgeist of the time of their development. Today, it seems unlikely that the current predominant therapies could offer as strong a justification for privileged communications and confidentiality as the psychodynamic therapies of years past. If we consider the case of Normita in Chapter Six—which reflects an actual and frequent situation in a community—involving family members in the work of the spirit-mediums at spiritist centers would seem to work against any need to restrict access of information between healer and client.

Although statutes and ethical standards may promote compliance with the dominant society's values and beliefs, they may operate in opposition to a minority culture's values and beliefs. We do not advocate disregarding these standards when dealing with Latinos. However, we caution practitioners to be aware of the values and beliefs of varied Latino cultures. If specific accommodations to current clinical practice can be made without breaching extant statutes and ethical standards of our mental health professions, we should be willing to make these accommodations.

How Clinical Practice Is Influenced by the Exosystem

Until recently, most practitioners did not think of community contexts as domains for intervention or areas that must be considered when developing and guiding interventions at the microsystemic or mesosystemic levels. In this section, we consider how the community is implicated in the ways in which youth and adult subcultures are created, in the way certain experiences are transmitted across generations, in the ethnic identities that youths assume and espouse, in spiritual practices, and in economic conditions.

Conflict Between Subcultures

As already mentioned, one of our objections to teaching "the facts you need to know about Latinos" is that this approach more often than not leads to stereotyping because it ignores intragroup variations. Each ethnic group contains many subcultures. Practitioners need to explore with their client the relevant subcultures in that youth's life, those to which the youth feels he or she belongs, and those with which the youth's preferred subculture conflicts. The following cases are relevant.

> Chepito, a fifteen-year-old Mexican American boy, is the prototypical *cholo*—member of a subculture of the streets. He uses all the right slang. He is sure to intersperse the necessary slang terms like *ese* (hey, you), *pinche* (subservient), and *puta madre* (whore mother) in his conversations with his homeboys. He has just the right hair bob and hand gestures. He dresses in white sleeveless undershirts and black extra-wide-leg pants slung down low around his hips to expose his boxer shorts.
>
> Chepito lives in the projects of East Los Angeles. His father, an abusive alcoholic, abandoned the family two years earlier to live with another woman. His mother works for low wages with poor benefits in the highly exploitative

garment industry. The small world of his neighborhood and his fellow *cholos* and *cholas* provide Chepito with a sense of self-worth and support that contrasts with the sense of devaluation and failure he gets at school and his estrangement from his family, whom he believes want him to be a "throwback" to the way his mother remembers youths raised in Mexico. In his darkest moments, Chepito writes intense rap songs that express his existential angst; no one but his "homies" knows that he has this creative streak. Indeed, his homies look up to Chepito. In his self-presentation and his rap, they see an intense and charismatic youth who cannot live life passively. But his sartorial splendor and well-practiced *cholo* demeanor are a great embarrassment to his mother, and he is the object of quiet ridicule from diverse groups of preppies, surfers, goths, and others at the large public school he attends. Chepito strives to live up to the idealized image of the *cholo* that has been created by a subculture that has long existed and that he has recently entered. The California *cholos* of Chepito's generation are not unlike the *pachucos* of the 1940s.

Jessie, a sixteen-year-old Cuban–Mexican American girl, attends a private high school with a very small ethnic minority student population. She is outgoing, self-assured, and very popular with her peers, and she excels academically. Her circle of friends is culturally and economically diverse. Her middle-class parents work hard to provide Jessie with opportunities they didn't have when they were growing up. Both parents work: Mother is an elementary school teacher and Father is a counselor for at-risk youth in a church-affiliated social service agency. The family lives in a safe, ethnically mixed middle-class neighborhood. This summer, Jessie will go on a trip to Europe with her class—another opportunity that her parents never had. She identifies herself as Hispanic and does not speak Spanish. She enjoys her mother's Cuban cooking and some but not all of her parents' Cuban and Mexican traditions and celebrations. Like her peers at school, she likes alternative rock music. Jessie's rapid assimilation into mainstream society may be attributed in part to her parents' efforts to broaden her experiences beyond those they had as youngsters.

Other than being Latino, Chepito and Jessie have little in common. Chepito's *cholo* subculture offers him some immediate benefits that are likely to keep him severed both from his traditional Latino subculture and the dominant mainstream. To the outside observer, his future looks bleak; it is difficult to appreciate his values, beliefs, and attitudes. To his mother, Chepito is the cross she must bear, at once cherishing it and resenting it for the pain it causes. To his teachers, Chepito is an incorrigible gangster destined for academic failure and delinquency. Because he has joined a subculture that separates him from traditional Mexican culture and from other youth subcultures in his community, no one beyond his equally isolated homies will ever recognize his creativity and potential for leadership. In contrast, Jessie's future is very promising. Yet her success may come at the expense of losing her Cuban and Mexican cultures if she continues to assimilate to the majority culture.

Chepito's and Jessie's development is influenced by others beyond peers, family, and school. It is influenced by the subcultures that interact with their personal contexts. Chepito has grown up in poverty, with an abusive father, in a violent neighborhood. Jessie has been spared the environmental stressors that Chepito has experienced. She has lived a "protected" life that has allowed her to optimize her potential in the dominant society.

Transgenerational Experiences

In the past few years, increasing attention has been given to historical trauma in the lives of children, as in the cases of Jewish children of survivors of the Holocaust and of American Indian children whose parents and many generations before them lived through oppression, prejudice, and efforts to eradicate their cultures (tribes relocated to different parts of the country or children sent to boarding schools far from their reservations, for example). Similarly, many children of Guatemalan and Salvadoran immigrants are the inheritors of the trauma suffered by their parents and grandparents before their emigration. In this type of transgenerational traumatization, the exosystemic contexts that must be explored are separated by time and location and do not include the individual.

Traumatization is but one event that can be experienced across generations. Other experiences, both positive and negative, can have profound and lasting effects on the progeny of those who have lived through them. Although attending to negative transgenerational experiences sheds light on important processes that often were ignored in mental health practice, attending to positive transgenerational effects can help tap into aspects that can inform prevention efforts and aid in developing more effective interventions. One such positive phenomenon is the importance of a person's name and the legacy attached to it. Although this is common to many cultures, it is important to appreciate its relevance in Latino cultures.

Ramon Samaniego is a seventeen-year-old Mexican American teenager who is the oldest of six siblings and attends an urban Catholic high school. He is likely to be named valedictorian of his class. He has been an exemplary student and an outstanding role model for his peers. Ramon's motivation to excel and to do well derive in large part from his deep sense of responsibility and loyalty to his family. Ramon feels intense pride about his last name and his heritage. The name Samaniego is well respected in the village where Ramon's father Miguel grew up. During a recent summer trip with his family to the village, Ramon's father talked proudly to one of his friends about Ramon's accomplishments. His father's friend told Miguel in Ramon's presence: *"De tal palo, tal astilla. ¡Que espera, Don Miguel, es un Samaniego!"* ("From such a stick, such a splinter. What do you expect, Don Miguel, he is a Samaniego!")

Thus, Ramon is aware of the responsibility of living up to this expectation and the necessity not to bring shame to the family name. He understands that individual failure or shameful behavior will tarnish not only his reputation but also that of his immediate family and that of generations that follow. When Ramon has felt overburdened by the expectations of his father and the family, he draws solace from the story he has heard many times, and in many versions, about his great grandfather, Don Manuel.

By all accounts, Don Manuel was an exceptional man of admirable character and unblemished dignity who, during the Mexican Revolution, fought hard for "the cause" without ever getting tainted or corrupted or resorting to the savagery that often accompanies battle. The villagers he led in battle considered him their leader and loved and admired him; his wife would talk about his love for and devotion to his children; and his children would talk about their parents' relationship, a union of two strong-willed individuals whose love for each other endured many trials and tribulations. Don Manuel's life was never an easy one, yet he lived his life with grace and integrity.

The expectation that Ramon will live up to the family name both guides and directs Ramon, and when Ramon gets married, it is hoped pride in the family name will guide and direct his children.

These transgenerational experiences connect individuals across several generations. "Who a person is" is not just a product of what a person does in his or her lifetime. Personal identity extends from the individual's predecessors to successors. Individual accomplishments are subordinated to collective achievements of a family over many generations because the individual is one link in a long and intricate chain. An individual can feel pressure to "live up" to the family name and bring honor to the family, but this connectedness also can bring support and solace as well as a sense of life's deeper meaning. It is likely that the intense pride in and loyalty to a gang and its name, which is observed in Latino gangs, arise because of a breakdown in the family that severs the sense of shared transgenerational experiences. The gang and its name come to supplant the family and family-name pride that has been lost. Thus, the threat to a secure sense of meaning in life that extends beyond one's immediate accomplishments, especially when these are lacking, may be one of the reasons some Latino youths are attracted to gangs.

Awareness of both positive and negative transgenerational experiences can guide a contextually oriented practitioner to intervene at the exosystemic level. In working with Latino youth who do not seem to react to motivators that practitioners often tap into, it can be useful to explore with the youth and family issues pertaining to dignifying the family in a transgenerational way by the actions in which one preserves the honor of the family name in living one's life. If therapists explore with a youth and family their history and identify remarkable ancestors who can serve as inspirations and ideal figures against which a youth can judge his or her own conduct, it may lead to powerful exosystemic interventions.

Ethnic Identity

Martha Bernal and George Knight state that ethnic identity is determined by two processes: *enculturation*, which refers to the socialization of youth in their culture of origin, and *acculturation*, which refers to the process of adapting to the host culture.[19] Ethnic identity as the outcome of these two processes involves the exosystem in that an individual is influenced by some contexts in which he is not a direct participant. Bernal and Knight describe five components of ethnic identity: *ethnic self-identification* (what a youth calls himself or herself); *ethnic constancy* (the awareness that ethnicity will stay the same over time and situation); *ethnic role behaviors* (involvement in cultural practices of the ethnic group); *ethnic knowledge* (understanding of the cultural practices of the ethnic group); and *ethnic preferences and feelings* (preferences and affinity for members of the same ethnic group or for cultural practices of the same ethnic group). They suggest that the abilities necessary to manifest these behaviors do not develop fully until about eight to ten years of age.

Bernal and Knight contend that a secure ethnic identity may be a buffer against prejudice and its deleterious effects. As we mentioned earlier, building the ethnic identity of a Mexican American or a Puerto Rican may be an important goal of therapy. To do this, the therapist must make an adequate assessment of the exosystem. For example, does the youth live in a community that is predominantly of the same ethnic group, a mix of ethnic groups, or European American? How have the communities in which the youth has lived influenced how he or she sees himself or herself with respect to ethnic identity? With whom does the youth identify? How does the youth feel about his ethnic membership, the ethnic identity of his parents and siblings, and the ethnic identity of his peers? How strong is the youth's ethnic identity, and what features of the family, school, neighborhood, and peer group enhance or weaken ethnic identity?

Living Up to Imposed Labels

Ethnic identity is a difficult construct to assess because culture is constantly changing and new subcultures are being created. A youth must deal with both the stereotypes and expectations of the host community and those of the specific community (for example, the Mexican American community). In the case of Chepito, it may be difficult to appreciate fully his sense of ethnic identity without understanding his relationship to the community in which he lives. To his Mexican parents and relatives, he may be a boy who has rejected traditional Mexican culture and allowed himself to be negatively influenced by an undesirable "American" subculture. To his teachers, he may be a recalcitrant youth who is just "like other Mexicans" who do not want to acculturate to the host community. To his homeboys, he may be a great example of how to be a Southern Californian *cholo* and live *la vida loca*. Chepito might feel that he is trying to break away from his Mexican roots while also refusing to join the *gabacho* (European American) world by staying in the *cholo* subculture. Contextually oriented practitioners must be cognizant of the subcultures in the communities in which they work, and how these subcultures affect their young clients.

Collective Terms and Ethnic Labels

In Chapter One we discussed the problem of trying to live up to imposed collective terms such as *Hispanic* or *Latino*. Latino youths, like other minorities, live with many expectations that arise from imposed labels. From a sociopolitical standpoint, the use of collective terms appears to be yet another manifestation of the assimilationist orientation of the American melting-pot ideology. Collective terms imposed by the host community may represent one step in the process of giving up one's ethnic identity—for example, going from Mexican American to Hispanic to American. From an exosystemic perspective, communities establish both implicitly and explicitly certain stereotypes and expectations about collective classifications. A Mexican American youth may have a good idea of what it is to be *Mexican* but a poor idea of what it is to be *Latino*. To understand his "Mexicanness," he can look to his family, his Mexican and Mexican American peers, and the communities of Mexicans and Mexican Americans in the region in which he lives. But to whom does he look to define what being *Latino* means? What will be gleaned from looking at Mexican Americans, Cuban Americans, Puerto Ricans, South Americans, and Central Americans in an effort to define "Latino-ness"? When a girl says she is Latina, what does she mean? How *homogenized*—to use Oboler's term[20]—will this self-identity be? Does a strong self-identity as a Latina have the same buffering effect as a strong Mexican American self-identity?

In the absence of research findings to guide clinical practice, a contextually oriented practitioner must attempt to understand each client's self-perception as it pertains to both ethnic-specific and collective labels, and appreciate how the client's ethnic identity either buffers potential stressors, like prejudice, or exacerbates a sense of inadequacy or vulnerability and stress.

Religion and Latino Communitarian Spirituality

With the exception of pastoral counseling, mental health practice has generally avoided the role of religion in people's lives, despite the important role it plays in the lives of many. One survey on the religiosity of psychotherapists found that whereas 33 percent of clinical psychologists reported that religious faith was the most important influence in their lives, 72 percent of the general population considered religious faith as the most important influence in their lives.[21] Some have argued that psychology's separation from religion or metaphysical issues has been based on a positivist view of science that is outmoded.[22] Stanton L. Jones has argued that there is no impermeable barrier between religion and science; he asserts that there needs to be "a greater awareness in the psychological community of the importance and pervasiveness of religious beliefs and commitments to the scientific and professional objectives of contemporary psychology."[23] This perspective in psychology, although still a minority perspective, represents yet another change that is conducive to contextually oriented psychological intervention. It is difficult to imagine how a contextually oriented practitioner could ignore something as important and pervasive in the lives of clients as religion and spirituality. In the case of Latinos, religion and spirituality—which we discussed in Chapter Three from a microsystemic perspective—often exerts a powerful influence when considered at the exosystemic level.

It is beyond the scope of this chapter to discuss the many ways in which religion and spirituality affect Latinos, so we will focus on one example. In Chapter Three we described the communitarian spirituality that Ana María Díaz-Stevens believes characterizes the spirituality practiced by Latinos in the United States.[24] This type of spirituality helps Latinos define themselves as an ethnic group by creating and reaffirming social bonds in a particular community. The importance of this type of spirituality is often ignored by practitioners who may view spirituality as out of the bounds of psychological intervention. However, as we noted in Chapter Six, from a contextual perspective, communitarian spirituality may represent an important source of support for Latino youths and their families. Reconnecting a Latina youth who is struggling with depression, a sense of isolation and hopelessness, and substance abuse to a spiritual group may offer her an avenue for reestablishing positive social bonds and developing a deeper sense of meaning in life.

Poverty and Interventions

In Chapter One, we noted that about 20 percent of Latino families live in poverty, twice as many as non-Latino families; the median income for Latinos is approximately $25,000, or $10,000 less than for all other Americans. Poverty is an exosystemic process that directly affects the developing individual. For example, children who live in poverty have lower IQ scores than children who do not live in poverty, and early intervention has beneficial effects on IQ scores regardless of risk factors such as low birth weight, parental unemployment, maternal depression, and teenage motherhood.[25] Social risk—defined as poverty or single-parent families—has been found to be associated with behavioral difficulties among preschoolers, regardless of whether it is accompanied by biological risk factors such as low birth weight, neurosyphilis, or sickle-cell anemia.[26] Elementary-school-age children living in disadvantaged neighborhoods experience more stressful life events.[27] Stressful life events have been found to be associated with higher levels of concurrent aggression and to predict increases in aggression one year later; life transitions and exposure to violence have been found to predict concurrent aggression.[28] Long-term poverty has been found to predict children's academic performance (decreases in math and reading scores) and antisocial behavior problems.[29] Premature, low birth weight babies born into poverty have been shown to have a very poor prognosis for functioning in all areas of development. Nevertheless, those raised in a setting with three or more protective factors (such as low density in the home, a safe area to play, responsiveness of the parent, and so on) and those who participated in a multisite infant development intervention program more often showed early signs of resiliency than children who did not have the protective factors or participate in the program.[30]

When working with poor Latino youths and their families, it is important to examine both the potential deleterious effects of poverty as well as ways of mitigating these deleterious effects (increasing protective factors in the home environment, for example). A contextually oriented practitioner might explore ways to help the family improve its financial and living situation. The practitioner might link up a single parent with a job training program, with a vocational education program, or with a case manager who could help the family find better, lower-density, safer housing. The practitioner might look for special programs for the child that capitalize on strengths the child already has (such as a neighborhood summer swimming program or a citywide mentoring program that links professionals—such as writers or computer engineers—with youth who might develop an interest in those professions). In addition, the practitioner might help the parents improve their responsiveness to and monitoring of their children, bring into the home more enriching learning materials, and provide the children with a wider variety of experiences in and outside the home. These efforts might be accomplished through a team consisting of the therapist, a case manager, and a behavior management specialist who visits the home regularly at the therapist's direction. Or the therapist may connect the parents to parent support, advocacy, church, or community groups that can help them develop these protective mechanisms.

Conclusion

This chapter has provided a broad overview of selected aspects of the exosystem that might be considered when assessing and treating Latino youths and their families. Appreciating how the exosystem is involved in the life of a Latino youth, both positively and negatively, can help direct the contextually oriented practitioner in selecting and implementing interventions. For the contextually oriented practitioner, the crucial issue is how the Latino youth can develop optimally within his "natural" environment (his local world). Thus, an integral aspect of the task of psychological intervention is to determine the youth's participation in contexts beyond the personal and to plan how the youth can derive maximum benefit for a successful life in those contexts.

Endnotes

1. S. W. Henggeler and C. M. Borduin, *Family Therapy and Beyond: A Multisystemic Approach to Treating the Behavior Problems of Children and Adolescents* (Pacific Grove, Calif.: Brooks/Cole, 1990); S. W. Henggeler,

G. B. Melton, and L. A. Smith, "Family Preservation Using Multisystemic Therapy: An Effective Alternative to Incarcerating Serious Juvenile Offenders," *Journal of Consulting and Clinical Psychology, 60*(6) (1992): 953–961; J. Szapocznik and others, "The Evolution of Structural Ecosystemic Theory for Working with Latino Families," in *Psychological Interventions and Research with Latino Populations,* ed. J. G. Garcia and M. C. Zea (Needham Heights, Mass.: Allyn & Bacon, 1997), 166–190.

2. R. M. Friedman, "Restructuring of Systems to Emphasize Prevention and Family Support," *Journal of Clinical Child Psychology, 23* (supplement, 1994): 40–47; R. M. Friedman, K. Kutash, and A. J. Duchnowski, "The Population of Concern: Defining the Issues," in *Children's Mental Health: Creating Systems in a Changing Society,* ed. B. A. Stroul (Baltimore: Paul H. Brooks, 1996); R. M. Friedman, "Services and Service Delivery Systems for Children with Serious Emotional Disorders: Issues in Assessing Effectiveness," in *Evaluating Mental Health Services: How Do Programs for Children "Work" in the Real World?* ed. C. T. Nixon and D. A. Northrup (Thousand Oaks, Calif.: Sage, 1997).

3. K. Hoagwood, "Introduction to the Special Section: Issues in Designing and Implementing Studies in Non–Mental Health Care Sectors," *Journal of Clinical Child Psychology, 23*(2) (1994): 114–115.

4. J. C. Meyers, "Financing Strategies to Support Innovations in Service Delivery to Children," *Journal of Clinical Child Psychology, 23* (supplement, 1994): 48–54.

5. J. H. Hanley, "Use of Bachelor-Level Psychology Majors in the Provision of Mental Health Services to Children, Adolescents, and Their Families," *Journal of Clinical Child Psychology, 23* (supplement, 1994): 55–58.

6. D. Cicchetti and M. Lynch, "Toward an Ecological/Transactional Model of Community Violence and Child Maltreatment: Consequences for Children's Development," *Psychiatry, 56* (1993): 95–118.

7. K. Hodges, *CAFAS Manual for Training Coordinators, Clinical Administrators, and Data Managers, 1997* (available from Kay Hodges, Ph.D., 2140 Old Earhart Road, Ann Arbor, MI 48105; fax 734/769–1424).

8. Hodges, *CAFAS Manual,* 1–1.

9. E. M. Koppitz, *The Bender-Gestalt Test for Young Children* (Philadelphia: Grune & Stratton, 1963); E. M. Koppitz, *The Bender-Gestalt Test for Young Children,* vol. 2, *Research and Application, 1963–1973* (Philadelphia: Grune & Stratton, 1973); P. Lacks, *Bender-Gestalt Screening for Brain Dysfunction* (New York: Wiley Interscience, 1984).

10. K. E. Berry, *Developmental Test of Visual-Motor Integration* (River Grove, Ill.: Follet, 1974).

11. A. L. Benton, *The Revised Visual Retention Test* (New York: Psychological Corporation, 1974).
12. J. Knitzer, *Unclaimed Children: The Failure of Public Responsibility to Children and Adolescents in Need of Mental Health Services* (Washington, D.C.: Children's Defense Fund, 1982).
13. B. A. Stroul and R. M. Friedman, *A System of Care for Severely Emotionally Disturbed Children and Youth* (Washington, D.C.: Georgetown University Child Development Center, CASSP Technical Assistance Center, 1986).
14. R. M. Friedman, "Services and Service Delivery Systems for Children with Serious Emotional Disorders: Issues in Assessing Effectiveness," in *Evaluating Mental Health Services: How Do Programs for Children "Work" in the Real World?* ed. C. T. Nixon and D. A. Northrup (Thousand Oaks, Calif.: Sage, 1997).
15. M. C. Roberts and M. Hinton-Nelson, "Models for Service Delivery in Child and Family Mental Health," in *Model Practices in Service Delivery in Child and Family Mental Health,* ed. M. C. Roberts (Hillsdale, N.J.: Erlbaum, 1996).
16. "Factsheet: Comprehensive Community Mental Health Services for Children Program." [http://www.mentalhealth.org/child/ccmhse.htm], Feb. 12, 1996.
17. "Factsheet," p. 2.
18. "Factsheet," pp. 1–2.
19. M. E. Bernal and G. P. Knight, "Ethnic Identity of Latino Children," in *Ethnic Identity: Formation and Transmission Among Hispanics and Other Minorities,* ed. M. E. Bernal and G. P. Knight (New York: State University of New York Press, 1993).
20. S. Oboler, *Ethnic Labels, Latino Lives: Identity and the Politics of (Re)Presentation in the United States* (Minneapolis: University of Minnesota Press, 1995).
21. A. Bergin and J. Jensen, "Religiosity of Psychotherapists: A National Survey," *Psychotherapy, 27* (1990): 3–7.
22. S. L. Jones, "A Constructive Relationship for Religion with the Science and Profession of Psychology: Perhaps the Boldest Model Yet," *American Psychologist, 49*(3) (1994): 184–199; W. Bevan, "Contemporary Psychology: A Tour Inside the Onion," *American Psychologist, 46*(5) (1991): 475–483; W. O'Donohue, "The (Even) Bolder Model: The Clinical Psychologist as Metaphysician-Scientist-Practitioner," *American Psychologist, 44*(12) (1989): 1460–1468.
23. Jones, "A Constructive Relationship."
24. A. M. Díaz-Stevens, *Latino Popular Religiosity and Communitarian Spirituality,* Program for the Analysis of Religion Among Latinos (PARAL), Occasional Paper no. 4 (1996).

25. F. R. Liaw and J. Brooks-Gunn, "Cumulative Familial Risks and Low-Birthweight Children's Cognitive and Behavioral Development," *Journal of Clinical Child Psychology, 23*(4) (1994): 360–372.

26. C. D. Adams, N. Hillman, and G. R. Gaydos, "Behavioral Difficulties in Toddlers: Impact of Sociocultural and Biological Risk Factors," *Journal of Clinical Child Psychology, 23*(4) (1994): 373–381.

27. B. K. Attar, N. G. Guerra, and P. H. Tolan, "Neighborhood Disadvantage, Stressful Life Events, and Adjustment in Urban Elementary-School Children," *Journal of Clinical Child Psychology, 23*(4) (1994): 391–400.

28. Attar, Guerra, and Tolan, "Neighborhood Disadvantage."

29. E. F. Dubow and M. F. Ippolito, "Effects of Poverty and Quality of the Home Environment on Changes in the Academic and Behavioral Adjustment of Elementary-School-Age Children," *Journal of Clinical Child Psychology, 23*(4) (1994): 401–412.

30. R. H. Bradley and others, "Contribution of Early Intervention and Early Caregiving Experiences to Resilience in Low-Birthweight, Premature Children Living in Poverty," *Journal of Clinical Child Psychology, 23*(4) (1994): 425–434.

Chapter Eight

Culture: The Pervasive Context

The Legacy of Conquest is over and we must adjust—some,
But never compromise your beliefs or customs.
PLACIDO VASQUEZ JR.

In the preceding chapters, we explored selected problems and
types of distress experienced by youths in the larger Latino populations in the United States embedded in situations encountered
within microsystemic (personal), mesosystemic (linked), and exosystemic (community) contexts. For the sake of simplicity we also
described our approach to intervening in problems at each of these
contextual levels, even though we also advanced the notion that all
the contexts are interwoven in an individual's life and experiences.
Although we have described the macrosystemic level as integral to
our contextual approach, this chapter's content is somewhat different from that of the preceding chapters. Culture contextualizes
every aspect of human life, including behavior problems, distress,
and development. If contexts are seen to be interwoven, we might
say that the daily activities, or cultural practices, are the woof of a
youth's life-fabric (a weaving-in-process), whereas development is
the warp. Culture is the overall design: it provides meanings associated with daily activities.

Interventions at the macrosystemic level might by analogy lead
to new designs for cultural practices for a segment, or for a whole
ethnic group, or even for a society at large. This actually occurs when
members of a minority group acculturate to the majority culture (for

example, when Latino immigrant youths adopt ideas, meanings, and associated behavior patterns encountered in mainstream North American society). However, change may lead to stress as a result of feelings of alienation from both one's own group and a chosen other social group—as may happen, for example, if a youth rejects his Mexican immigrant peers but then is not accepted by peers in the European American group he has chosen because he is dark complected or expresses himself in accented English.[1] Consequently, interventions might focus on a social institution or the society at large and have the goal of assisting the immigrant youth's integration in a less stressful way. For example, an entire school system might incorporate teaching materials and experiences that view Mexican culture in a positive light into its curriculum plans with the intent of promoting an understanding of immigrant youths' experience in a new country. Or interventions might consist of far-reaching political and economic changes, such as those accomplished through social engineering or new social philosophies. For example, change might be accomplished by legislating and institutionalizing ways generally to improve schools and curricula that serve Latino children, thereby expanding their opportunities to attain middle class and professional status, which in time will assist them in overcoming discriminatory attitudes. Or a public policy might be advocated in which the concept of race as an index of social stratification and inherent measure of an individual's or group's worth and capacities is eliminated.

Cultural Orientations

In Chapter Two we noted that a renowned anthropologist, A. I. Hallowell, long ago specified that the relationship between the self and its context is referenced by a "culturally constituted behavioral environment" that considers the "properties and adaptational needs of the organism in interaction with the external world as constituting the actual behavioral field."[2] According to Hallowell, culture provides five basic orientations as conditions for self-awareness:

- *Self-orientation:* Expressed through names, personal pronouns, gender identity, sexual orientation, and so on

- *Object orientation:* Concepts, classification, and attributes of objects related to the self, such as other persons, other-than-human persons (like God or spirits), materials, tools, and natural events
- *Spatiotemporal orientation:* Locating selves in time and space
- *Motivational orientation:* Goals that satisfy needs and dispositions toward activities
- *Normative orientation:* Values, ideals, standards, system of morality

We will touch on each of these areas, giving specific examples for selected Latino cultures. We note that there can be considerable intragroup variation within Latino cultures, much as there is between Latino cultures. However, some general cultural orientations—such as acknowledging the Spanish language as a mother tongue—are widely shared among Latino cultures in the United States. Cultural orientations can be described as shared patterns established by the need for cooperation, communication, and the passing on of tradition. However, cultures as patterns of guiding ideas are actualized in the interactions and activities of people in particular social groups. The relationship between cultural orientations and how cultures are actualized in local worlds leads to many orientations being changeable, negotiable and, at times, contested.

In concert with many anthropologists and cultural psychologists, we believe that culturally specific orientations toward the self and other selves have substantial continuity across an individual's life span and act as indices or points of reference in myriad activities. For example, the age or behavior that is certified as mature and responsible in a male deemed old enough to marry, and the age at which or behavior by which a female is considered qualified to do so, are sanctioned by cultural orientations toward gender. They are also supported by concepts and meanings associated with a developmental stage that might be termed "adult," "mature," or something similar, and by standards for conduct in and ideals about marriage. In instances involving immigration, acculturation, or culture change, there are often competing cultural orientations that may lead to conflicting ideals, values, and standards being held by different family members who may experience distressing ambivalence over the differences between what they feel is appropriate behavior and what their parents or peers advocate.

This chapter will review aspects of cultural orientations that affect youths' development and are significant in problems experienced by Latino families and youths. We feel it is especially important to explore how ideas, values, and perspectives interact with the ongoing process of development in youths and constitute their lifescapes. Although we briefly described aspects of cultural orientations as a backdrop to understanding Latinos in Chapter One and later referred to them in the cases and proposed interventions described in earlier chapters, in this chapter we will paint a broader cultural landscape to complement the less encompassing levels of context that those chapters examined. We will also elaborate on the effects of cultural processes that are particularly relevant to Latinos—such as self-identification and ethnic identification, socialization, immigration, and acculturation—on Latino youths' problem behaviors and emotional distress. Each section explores how an understanding of orientations toward the self and toward others and cultural processes affects the task of formulating and contextualizing interventions.

Self-Orientation: Who Am I?

When working with youths, self-orientation is often a central aspect of interventions. For Latino youths, it is particularly important to considering gender and social identities to address both problems and solutions.

Gender Identity

The self-concept among Latino youth includes, among others, two important dimensions that are central to our approach to contextual interventions: gender identity and social identity. Although there are many theories of gender identity, gender schema theory serves our approach in that it links both environmental factors and individual cognitive processing, and it emphasizes social learning within particular contexts.[3] Gender schema theory looks at gender identity from both social and individual perspectives. It proposes that persons become gender-typed (initiating the acquisition of self-concepts, preferences, behavior patterns, and so on) perhaps as early as three to five years of age. Latino cultures strongly differentiate between the sexes and socialize children for specifically identified male or female gender roles. There seems to be little ambiguity regarding gender identification of very small children. For example, in the poorer rural areas and some urban areas of Puerto Rico and the Dominican Republic where diapers are not used, male toddlers walk about with only a small shirt covering their upper bodies. In contrast, the genitals of female babies are invariably covered.

This is the initiation of a number of complex gender role patterns that address the need to protect women (young girls especially) from the ever-watchful, sexualized interests of men. Girls and young women are mandated to maintain an aloofness from all expressions of male sexuality. Through a series of developmentally related idealized patterns of behavior for each of the sexes (for example, preadolescent and older boys are much freer to roam the streets, whereas girls must stay close to home), this leads to the ideal that women should protect their virginity until married. In contrast, young men are encouraged (even pushed) to have early sexual experience with "loose" women whom they should not marry. These attitudes are promoted by parent behaviors that dichotomously type youth into male and female, and these attitudes become normalized points of orientation about gender identity for children as they develop. The widespread custom among Puerto Ricans of calling very small children *mamita* (little mother) and *papito* (little father) illustrates the predilection for early gender typing.

Literature on Latino culture is replete with stereotypes. There is a considerable amount of debate in the literature on Latino cultures about the validity of the stereotypical patterns of male "machismo" and female "marianismo."[4] These patterns describe culturally typed and selected personality attributes that provide distinct images of males and females. The stereotype of Latina women is that they are and should be groomed to be submissive to males, home- and family-centered, focused on nurturing others to the point of self-sacrifice, as chaste as possible (even within marriage), and loyal and faithful to a mate for life, even holding in distress in the face of his peccadillos or abuse. In direct contrast, the stereotype of Latino males holds that they dominate women and children, very strongly assert their needs and desires, and are highly sexual and even predatory. It has been said that men are "traditionally socialized to validate their masculinity through control, power, and competition."[5] Studies of men who are physically abusive or abuse alcohol or drugs conclude that these problems are related to these men having been socialized in a traditional way.[6]

Apart from the very valid criticisms that these stereotypical images of male and female gender roles do not take social class, acculturation, or regional differences into account and are clearly overgeneralized, it is also obvious that they are negatively toned depictions. Positive versions of these stereotypes might depict idealized gender roles in the family. For example, women most frequently take care of the household and family affairs and, in many places in the United States, are the brokers between the family and the community. Men bear the responsibility for financial support, make major decisions (often in consultation with their spouses), and provide a sense of security and stability to the family. This division of roles is probably more frequent in an agrarian setting but appears much more rarely in the urban Latino populations in the United States where family life is deeply affected by employment opportunities for men and women and by economic goals, which in turn are affected by the vagaries of the economies of different cities and regions. Gender roles also are influenced by family structure and organization, variations that result from the presence of extended family, single motherhood, the adoption of new ideas as a result of acculturation, and level of education.[7]

The complexity of actual gender role behaviors in the family setting is described in a study of attitudes of Mexican American women and men.[8] Among first-generation respondents, more than one-half rejected a male-dominated family structure; among the second and third generations, even fewer endorsed it. Educational level plays a crucial role too: attempts of working-class women to establish a separate and autonomous identity strain marriage, as mentioned earlier in the case of Juan's parents.[9] Latina professional women may have less trouble being autonomous in work spheres but most complain about how they must maintain the heavy burdens of the household and child rearing in addition to putting careers on the back burner when they get home. (Of course, this is a general complaint of most professional women, regardless of ethnicity.) It is usually the case that women who are employed outside the home acquire a greater share of decision-making power within it, but this will play out differently depending on the spouses' orientation toward and expectations of marriage.

Male Gender Identity and Interventions

In Chapter Six we discussed the problem of recruiting Latino fathers into interventions such as family therapy or parent groups in the schools. Some have suggested that a "strong adherence to traditional male gender identity" may affect all aspects of the therapeutic process because these men avoid situations in which they might appear weak or no longer in control.[10] Latino men are also characterized as inhibiting emotional responses and being unaware of their feelings. These ideas are directed indiscriminately toward Latino men without cultural reference points. It has also been suggested that there may be a relationship between male adolescent endorsement of these masculine behaviors and problems of substance misuse, violence, delinquency, and sexual activity. However, this notion ignores the fact that non-Latino adolescents exhibit very similar behaviors, suggesting that important factors other than idealized gender patterns may be involved.

One pattern that may be very relevant to the gender concepts of Latino youths is that of early sexual activity without the use of contraception, but it is likely that this too varies by social class and acculturation level. Behavior in Latino male gangs might be described as "hypermasculinity" because it appears to mimic the stereotypical pattern, but we can inquire if this behavior is viewed as a way to gain "respect" (autonomy, social status, and so on) within communities that seem systematically to deny it to ethnic minority youths in general. As we have suggested in earlier chapters, this explanation of problem behavior in male youths should be verified through inquiries with the individual youth as a systematic part of an intervention strategy.

Social Identity and Ethnic Identity

Especially in activities with peers and in school, issues around social identity loom large in importance for Latino youth.[11] A review of these issues advocates a social identity approach to understanding group membership and its relationship to behavior with members of one's own or other groups.[12] Social identity theory specifies that our self-concept is partly developed through membership in our in-group. Whether that self-concept is positive or negative will depend on how we ourselves, and how others, view our group. Judgments of worth are determined by two processes: categorization of the groups and comparisons among them. A youth's behavior changes according to his social group's category, and according to in- or out-group judgments about its status. Social identity formation "becomes particularly salient in adolescence" as this is an identity-building and consolidating period.[13]

Within social identity, ethnic identity refers to a set of ideas that people have about their own ethnic group (ethnic self-concept), their closest social reference group, their behavioral preferences, and the way others perceive their group. The literature on ethnic identity among Latino children has its antecedents in formulations about racial identity among African Americans.[14] Descriptions of ethnic identity among Latinos generally focus on behavioral aspects— such as language, role behavior, preferences (for friends, foods, and so on)—and on ideational aspects, such as values, worldviews and self-views, and expressions of spirituality. These descriptions do not usually include race or racial identity. They do include both familial and nonfamilial socialization as well as children's cognitive development.[15]

Two aspects of ethnic identity are especially important when it comes to interventions with adolescents. First, ethnic identification is a *cognitive developmental process* in which awareness of ethnicity appears at five to ten years of age, ethnic self-identification at about seven years to ten, and constancy of ethnic identity at eight to ten years of age. By ten to fifteen years of age a cognitive developmental threshold has been reached and the process of ethnic self-identification inevitably runs in tandem with many other psychological and physical developmental processes. Second, ethnic identification is a *stage process,* with the timing and progression of ethnic identification differing among individuals and social groups. Some theorists suggest a three-stage model.[16] An early stage is characterized by lack of exploration of ethnicity and acceptance of the values and attitudes of the majority culture. Lack of exploration may be "diffuse" (that is, the individual may lack interest) or "foreclosed" (that is, the person's views are based on the opinions of others). A further stage in the process is the attempt to understand ethnicity from the individual's own perspective. At a final stage the individual may arrive at a clear sense of his or her ethnic identity. However, some youths remain confused and ambivalent into young adulthood. There are many reports of persons arriving at a firm sense of ethnic identity as part of their college experience, thanks to ethnic group activities. However, college attendance is fairly rare in the overall Latino population, as we indicated in Chapter One.

Social environmental factors (that is, cultural context) may be most significant in developing an ethnic identity. For example, when Latino youths experience discrimination frequently (as in some school or neighborhood situations), are confronted daily by negative stereotypes, and perceive that they are barred from full participation in the dominant group, they may early foreclose on their ethnic identity choice. However, this may also depend on earlier socialization and the parents' ethnic identification stage. For example, recently immigrated parents give their children a richer cultural background and more strongly influence their ethnic identity.[17] This is hardly surprising but speaks to the changing nature of ethnic group identification over generations of residency in the United States and also to variability within generations. It leads to an important question: Is the lack of certainty and clarity regarding ethnic identity associated with, or causally related to, behavior problems or emotional distress in youths?

As described in Chapter Seven, psychologists Martha Bernal and George Knight offer a general model of socialization for ethnic identity in Mexican American children that meets the criteria we have posed for a contextual approach.[18] They support an interactive perspective that shows that parents' socialization mediates between family background variables (use of Spanish or English language, value schema, and so on) and a youth's ethnic identity, which in turn is affected by socialization by nonrelatives (such as teachers, friends, and so on) and the social situations that the youth encounters outside the family. An ethnographic portrait of Mexican American youths in one California school describes how those who identify themselves as Chicano and reject both Mexican and mainstream American cultural orientations actively reject dominant culture values and experience school failure.[19] There are age and gender differences in the development of ethnic identity.

For example, Mexican American girls score higher than boys on more sophisticated measures of identity development, and younger adolescents usually score in the categories denoting the earlier stages of the process.

Problems in assessing ethnic identity include measuring ethnic identification as a process and understanding and assessing internal or behavioral outcomes related to the acquisition or constancy of ethnic identity. There are a number of recent studies of Mexican American youths but fewer explorations of social identity in other Latino groups. The role of phenotypical characteristics (such as skin color) is not dealt with extensively in the literature, but it is an especially important issue for ethnic identification among many Puerto Ricans and some Cubans, especially youths who are in close proximity to African American peers. As we mentioned in Chapter Three, skin color can also be an issue for youths of Mexican and Central American descent. Moreover, there are special issues around ethnic identity for Latino children adopted by parents from non-Latino cultures and in understanding the process of ethnic identification in youths from families of mixed ethnicity.[20]

Ethnic Identity and Interventions

In order to deal with school problems or other difficulties, it has been suggested that interventions directly address both ethnic identity and discrimination toward Latino youths by the dominant mainstream group.[21] In Chapter Four, we briefly described the innovative interventions by the Fordham University group of culturally adapted treatments for children and adolescents. In one intervention, Cuento Therapy, folktales are used to model behavior for Puerto Rican children in New York ages nine to thirteen, as a way to transmit cultural values and cultivate pride in their ethnic identity.[22] The Fordham group modifies traditional folktales to reflect values and skills judged useful in coping with the adopted U.S. environment.

An innovative group therapy modality for Mexican origin and Mexican American youths in the Southwest targeted issues of ethnic identity and discrimination after observing the role of generational conflict in families.[23] It was determined that the youths of Mexican descent, most in early adolescence, would not respond positively to a bicultural orientation. Southwestern societies frequently discriminate against children of Mexican descent because of their appearance and because of stereotypes about racial difference. Observation of group therapy process in this clinical sample corroborated the pretreatment observation that frequent interactions with peers, teachers, and the general public preclude comfort with a bicultural identity unless the youth appears Anglo—that is, has fair skin and speaks English fluently. A significant concern is this: How does the therapist decide whether to reinforce a "traditional" (Mexican) ethnic identity (whether or not adapted to the U.S. environment) or a bicultural identity? Studies of process within those interventions that target change in ethnic identity could answer this question, but they have yet to be carried out.[24] In the absence of process studies of treatment, therapists can sensitively inquire into this area for individual clients and their significant others.

Orientation Toward Persons and Objects: Who Are We?

Through modeling, observation, or direct instruction, from perhaps their earliest moments children learn idealized attitudes and behaviors preferred by parents or other caretakers that are often tied to the economic structure of a society and the economic niche occupied by the local group. For example, a common ideal in families across Latino subcultures is that of balance and harmony in their interactions as well as a heavy taboo on conflict and expressing aggression. Children are reared to depend on the family, with a clear priority on mutual obligations. Their individuality is fully recognized, even if frequently subordinated to family needs and goals. For many, this creates lifelong interdependence among members of the family of origin.

Themes for Behavior

The central and most emphasized themes for behavior are loyalty and respect for parents, which are mandated as correct, moral behavior. This mandate extends to elder siblings, grandparents, and aunts and uncles, as well as to surrogate parental authority figures outside the family. When it comes to preferred temperament and character, Puerto Rican mothers are clear that children must learn to show respect (*respeto*) and interest and warmth (*cariño*) toward others and maintain a calm mood (*tranquilidad*).[25] An in-depth description of socialization by Mexican American parents shows a special focus on their child's behaving appropriately in social situations, not being forward or assertive or infringing on the rights of others (*ser educado, decente*), and being highly respectful to older persons and those in authority.[26] Respect also connotes willingness to carry out the rules of sociability.[27] Although creative and individualistic behavior is highly prized, disruptive spontaneity can make parents uncomfortable if it encroaches on the dignity and respect owed to others. For poorer and less acculturated families, children have their place in an adult world rather than in a child-centered one.

In examining development and bilingualism, anthropological linguist Ana Celia Zentella vividly portrays socialization among Puerto Ricans in New York City by distinguishing between situation-versus child-centered processes.[28] Poorer families in Puerto Rico (and in New York) make few child-centered accommodations. The result is that children are almost never segregated from adults. Middle-class families display more child-centered behaviors. Children in less well-educated families generally learn by observation and imitation rather than by instruction, and "respect" means not interfering in adult activities at any time. Small children demonstrate their abilities and receive praise when they carry out assigned tasks rather than perform child-centered activities, such as athletics or games.

Many of the families studied in New York are descendants of families from rural barrios in Puerto Rico and appear to have many similar patterns of child rearing.[29] Even toddlers at one and a half years of age are praised for complying with instructions and carrying out tasks, such as cleaning up their messes or helping with a younger sibling. Very rarely do parents use a form of "baby language"; they routinely address even babies using adult linguistic forms. Latino families of Caribbean background seem more likely than other Latinos to encourage song and dance performances by their young children, but many Latinos have a deep appreciation for popular Latino music and encourage children to dance with others.

In the cultures of origin, even temporary physical or psychological separation from the nuclear family was not generally con-

sidered appropriate or desirable (and often not economically fea-
sible) until youths married or set up new households and families.
Only this arrangement conferred full adult status. However, among
immigrant families in the United States, a process of extrusion may
occur when children or teenagers are sent to live with extended
family members (grandparents or aunts and uncles) due to parents'
emigrating or moving, father's abandonment and mother's struggles to subsist, or because an adolescent's problem behaviors are so
disrupting that the family feels it cannot handle them. The receiving relatives are almost always in Mexico, Puerto Rico, or another
home country. One might call this last practice an *indigenous* contextual intervention because it intends an environmental change as
a remedy for a youth's problems. However, the result is often that
the youth feels at odds with both the culture of origin and U.S. environments as he or she first struggles to adjust to one and then
must revise orientations to adjust to the other. Child psychiatrist
Vincenzo Nicola calls the children of immigrants "changelings." He
recommends a special form of cultural family therapy in which "cultural encounters" between therapist and family focus intensively on
the cultural transitions that children and families undergo.[30]

Given the large number of troubled families in the United
States, Latino youths who have been psychologically extruded from
their homes because of problem behaviors and conflict with parents
but have no access to geographic solutions, and those youths who
feel they have failed to find respect and a "sense of dignity" at home
or school, often seek it on the streets. Anthropologist Philippe Bourgois's vivid ethnography of crack dealing in East Harlem is aptly ti-
tled *In Search of Respect,* referring to the importance of respect to an
individual's sense of uniqueness as a source of self-esteem.[31] Various
descriptions of Los Angeles gangs highlight street life as an alternative route to acquiring "honor" when other routes (education,
money, and higher social status) are perceived to be closed both
to the youths and their parents.[32]

A central aspect of the socialization process in the family involves drawing boundaries between those who are familiar and can
be trusted (*los de confianza*)—mainly family members and *compadres*
(godparents)—and those who are outsiders. Just as trust (*confianza*)
is extended to fictive kin through godparenting (*compadrazgo*), it is
also part of the idealized relationship among *manos* (street brothers)

or homeboys in the neighborhood. A public-private dichotomy affects interpersonal behavior on many levels. Among second-generation Mexican Americans and in other Latino cultures, a person's inner nature is considered sacrosanct, whereas his behavior is open for discussion and may even be the subject of gossip (*chisme*).[33] Social conformity is expected in many areas of life but not in one's inner life. This private-public distinction is based on attitudes about the prevalence of self-interest as a primary motivator and a view of the world as an unfriendly place, so that protecting one's private affairs is prudent.

Development and Problems

Recognizing that there are intergroup variations in Latino views on development, ideally a youth gradually takes on the responsibilities associated with adulthood, commonly believed to begin around fifteen years of age. There appears to be little recognition of a transition to be marked and attended to, or even an expectation of conflict with parents, whose main teaching instead is that they must be respected (with all the complex connotations that respect entails). One study found that Mexican American families have a significantly different response to puberty for boys than white families, in that Mexican American boys and their parents appear to relate to one another better.[34]

In our data from an intervention project in the Southwest, the poignant inability of large numbers of Mexican and Mexican American parents to relate to or understand the life experiences of their problem-behavior children and adolescents seems the result, in large part, of their having spent their early years in very different cultural settings and under very different conditions (whether in the United States or their country of origin). Immigrants and lower-income Mexican American parents are also forced to spend a great deal of time and energy on subsistence concerns.[35] This situation is exacerbated by the authoritarian pattern, however beneficent, in which most Mexican or Mexican American families relate to their children, whereby adolescents are usually not included in discussions of family problems if they are openly discussed at all. This exclusion extends to discussing the youth's problems with him or her. For the most part, in many Latino families, youths who are not nearing adulthood are much more often spoken *to* about problems than spoken *with*—at least until they are considered to be "responsible." As we have suggested in earlier discussions, in interventions undesirable behavior should be carefully assessed according to family definitions and perceptions. If parental judgments regarding such behavior brand the youth as irresponsible, then communication may be further closed down with the result that there is no possibility of effectively involving the youth.

Spatiotemporal Orientation: Where Are We in Space and Time?

A concern about who we are is closely associated with the notion of where we are in time and space. In this discussion, we reference the where by looking at the past in relation to the present, including the journeys from an ancestral place, either recently or in past generations, to the United States. The *ancestral place* or *home country* has very different meanings for each of the Latino cultures in the United States and these meanings vary across generations of residence here. Most first-generation immigrants from Mexico and the Dominican Republic seem to conserve their national identities, special cultural practices, and family connections in their original home regions. This is only partly true for Cubans; they conserve their national identity but have not had the same opportunity to visit and maintain a high degree of connection with the home country. Psychiatrist Pedro Ruiz describes how Cuban Americans have successfully adapted to life in the United States through an "integrational model" of adaptation in which their Cuban "heritage and traditions" have been preserved.[36] Immigrants from Central American countries who have fled terrorism also maintain their national identities but have relatively few contacts with their home countries and ambivalent feelings about preserving their general—as opposed to familial—relationship.

In contrast, some Mexican Americans identify as American and separate themselves from a Mexican national identity. But others, particularly those who have received higher education, have adopted an emergent identity as Chicanos, which "represents membership in a complementary community, as well as geographical and ideological loyalties."[37] Both popular and scholarly literatures frequently refer to Aztlán, a symbolic, ancestral home somewhere between Mexico and the United States, the "remains" of the Mexican territory annexed by the United States in the Treaty of Guadalupe in 1848.[38] A rap verse by a Mexican American teenager begins, "The Aztlán creation, a Latin nation." Recently, Chicanos have become more concerned with their relationship to Mexico.[39]

The situation of Puerto Ricans in the United States is quite different from that of the other Latino cultural groups. Because Puerto Ricans are U.S. citizens and move freely between the island and the mainland, they cannot be classified as immigrants in the usual sense. Although most identify strongly with their national culture, it is clear that their identity conflicts are widespread because Puerto Rican culture has emerged out of two colonial situations— the most recent lasting throughout the twentieth century—which fostered a sense of inferiority, a relative lack of self-determination and autonomy, and an indeterminacy of belonging.[40] Postmodern authors aptly describe the situation that is the result of political policies and the increasingly traveled two-way "bridge" between the island and the mainland, as the "translocality of Puerto Ricanness" or "Puerto Rican identity up in the air."[41]

The case is different for many second- and third-generation Puerto Ricans born in the United States. Some have not been to Puerto Rico and many marry non-Puerto Ricans and identify more as Latino Americans. Their relationship to the home country is more like that of the majority of children of European descent (although not as distanced), who do not focus on origins in a systematic or significant way. Complications of identity are brought about by racist ideas in the United States and affect those Puerto Rican children who have African features. Zentella, in describing socialization practices, notes that first-generation Puerto Rican parents in New York socialize their darker-skinned children to be aware of racial discrimination but also firmly insist that they identify as Puerto Ricans rather than as African Americans.[42]

Acculturation

There is general agreement that a consideration of acculturation— that is, cultural change as a result of continuous firsthand contact with the mainstream society—both as a process and as an attribute (such as the extent of involvement in and adoption of elements of U.S. culture) is essential to understanding, assessing, and intervening in behavioral and emotional problems.[43] In a review of studies to 1988 that link acculturation to mental health, medical sociologist Lloyd Rogler and his colleagues found that over half of the studies centered on Mexican Americans, less than a fourth focused on Puerto Ricans, a few looked at Cubans, and the rest examined a diversity of Latino groups. Among their conclusions was that the measurement of acculturation should be *orthogonal* rather than *unidimensional.* That is, level of involvement in U.S. society should not be assessed to mean a reduction of involvement in an immigrant's traditional culture.

The authors also examined hypotheses that acculturation, when measured unidimensionally, relates both positively and negatively to psychological distress—that is, highly acculturated persons may enjoy better mental health or very poor mental health, depending on the group examined. Biculturalism can also have positive and negative relationships to distress. Three studies showed a positive relationship between low psychological distress and biculturalism; other studies showed that higher acculturation predicted more alcohol and drug use, especially among first-generation Mexican Americans. The explanation for these phenomena favored by the authors was higher and unrealized aspirations among U.S.-born Mexican Americans in contrast to fewer aspirations among less acculturated persons, many of whom, as immigrants, perceive that they have satisfactorily improved their lives after migration. This is especially highlighted in the case of more acculturated Mexican American women, who are nine times more likely to misuse alcohol than those who are not as acculturated. This phenomenon may also reflect other things: that acculturation changes gender-role expectations or relationships, that marital relationships become more brittle and conflictual, that the women are less supported because extended family is absent, and that norms about women drinking alcohol change with the influence of mainstream U.S. culture.

Rogler and his colleagues ask for change in measuring the acculturation process toward considering the incorporation of aspects of more than one culture without corresponding decreases in either the original or adopted cultures. They also call for more detailed studies of the "complex dynamics of the process."[44] Relatively few studies examine the details of the process for Latino youths. A series of early studies explored the effect of acculturation on grade-school children of Mexican descent and concluded that second- and third-generation children lose their prosocial values in favor of competitive ones.[45] The authors speculate whether this is a result of adopting U.S. mainstream values or of the transition from a rural to an urban environment, the latter making demands for competitive behavior that Mexican American parents respond to in their socialization practices.

We described earlier some of the intergenerational conflicts between immigrant parents and their first-generation adolescent children. In a series of studies, sociologist William Vega and his colleagues chart the effects of acculturation as "strain" on Latinos in Dade County, Florida.[46] Among first-generation Latinos (culture unspecified but probably mostly Cuban American), teachers reported language conflicts, perceived discrimination, and perceptions of a closed society as very likely to affect school performance and lower educational aspirations. However, the authors reported that these conflicts were not evident in the youths' home settings. They suggested that youths born in this country are more sensitive than immigrant youths to definitions of the self that emerge out of interactions with majority youths at school. As mentioned earlier, Felix-Ortiz and Newcomb found a similar reaction among Mexican American youths in Southern California.[47]

Biculturalism and Interventions

As more recent work has denied the inevitability that one's culture of origin will disappear, researchers have instead explored *biculturalism,* which posits that the individual can become competent in two cultures without losing his or her cultural (or national) identity and not necessarily value one culture over another.[48] This perspective was described almost two decades ago by a University of Miami group that studies Cuban adolescents and their parents. Biculturalism is expressed in terms of the capacity to adopt behaviors from the new culture before acquiring its values. This perspective led to the development of a psychoeducational intervention called

Bicultural Effectiveness Training, which focused on coping with acculturation stresses that confront immigrant families and on diminishing conflict and distance between parents and adolescent children who are acculturating to the new society at different rates.[49] Researchers have consistently suggested that an integrated personal identity facilitates bicultural competence, defined as effectively managing life in two cultures.[50]

Despite the notion that biculturalism leads to better adjustment and less psychological distress, we must observe the ways in which youths become bicultural. The meanings they associate with particular behaviors or attitudes are a crucial part of the inquiry into the interactions between them and their contexts. Although a strong cultural identity may help youths to weather experiences of rejection in the cultures of origin or the new culture, many adolescents, either native-born or resident since their early years, have not yet developed strong personal and cultural identities. Therefore, they cannot risk reaching out to support groups in either culture and are unable to behave effectively in interpersonal relationships (by offering displays of respect or empathy or by being open to the worldviews and opinions of other youths).[51] To assess problems, each case must be understood in relation to the contexts targeted for intervention.

Bilingualism

There are complex issues around language and bilingualism among Latino youth related to psychosocial development and problem behavior as well as to interventions. However, most sociolinguistic studies that could inform us about language and cultural orientations of Latino youth have focused on educational issues, and many educators advocate linguistic assimilation. Examining bilingualism requires consideration of three things: a youth's actual proficiency in both languages, a youth's decisions regarding the use of a language in different settings, and what language means to the particular youth.[52] The few studies that have been conducted, such as those that document language conflicts as acculturative strains among Latino immigrant youth in educational settings in Florida, do not examine these different dimensions.[53]

Linguistic assimilation has been a preferred goal even in the few U.S. school systems that support bilingualism. This policy is blamed for the poor attitudes toward school that develop among many Latino youth.[54] As a very simple example, we might consider the phenomenon of anglicizing names for convenience when children are first enrolled in school. Names are very special in the Latino world. Last names are important because they indicate descent from both the father's and the mother's families. The tradition is to have one's father's family name followed by one's mother's; but this very frequently gets attentuated to one last name in the United States. Furthermore, most people are dubbed early in life with nicknames that point to a unique feature or are contractions of their names that connote affection and distinction. Not all of the features socially advertised are flattering: a lame child may be called *cojito* (little lame one), a dark-skinned child may be nicknamed *negrito* (little dark one). But these nicknames are also affectionate and intimate. Therefore, changing a child's name, no matter how much it facilitates biculturalism, may also symbolize a significant change in relationship to the child's family and a loss of the kinds of ancestral traditions we described in Chapter Seven.

We alluded earlier to the importance of understanding how particular children use each of the languages in their bilingual (or multilingual) repertoire. In the study of first- and second-generation Puerto Rican children in New York City we described earlier, it was apparent that differences between both English and Spanish as spoken in the homes of children or on the streets compared with how language is both spoken and used in the schools can lead to school failure. In addition, modes of teaching in the home versus the school may predispose children to poorer educational responses. For example, if the Puerto Rican child is expected to learn by observation and modeling at home but in school is constantly tested by verbal (and later written) queries, discouragement may set in before the child has had a chance to adapt to the change. Zentella suggests that more collaboration with youths and their parents in charting and understanding their use of both languages, as well as less insistence on standard forms of English and Spanish as the only languages used in the classroom, would encompass more of the bilingual youth's reality and lead to more successful learning.[55]

Bilingualism and Interventions

In this volume, we have advocated this same approach in intervening with bilingual youths and families. To begin with, understanding language use is crucial to an in-depth assessment of a youth's problems, activity settings, and situations (or to any diagnostic technique, as we suggested in Chapter Three). Apart from the understanding necessary to developing intervention strategies, there are a number of bilingual issues in treatment. What is the language of the deeper and more troubling emotions? What happens when a youth switches from one language to another? In the case of Jaime, for example, he would address the family therapist in English when he felt angry because he thought that his parents would not understand. By speaking in English, he could avoid confronting them in the session and publicly displaying a lack of respect. Bilingual youths play out all kinds of intergenerational conflict by switching to English, and some may hide their truer emotions by this means. In contrast, switching to formal Spanish may be used to detach the youth from the treatment process. Switching between English and Spanish is another process that should be observed and discussed with youths and their family members in a collaborative way. It may be viewed as integral to a youth's problems by others in his social contexts.

Motivational Orientation: What Should We Achieve?

Because of the largely agrarian and impoverished background of a large proportion of Latino immigrants in the United States (with the exception of some groups of Cubans), one explanation of the high value placed on family and interdependence is that they are a response to the challenges of survival and achievement of goals that motivated the move to the United States. Another view holds that separation from and loss of daily interactions with extended family members in the origin country promotes the contraction of the nuclear family unit, even though contacts with distant relatives may be frequent and continuous.

In the countries of origin, education beyond early adolescence for persons with low incomes is viewed as a highly desirable but distant ideal. Particularly among farmers and the working class, adolescence is not thought of as a unique developmental stage but rather as the first significant sign of a gradual and inevitable progression toward adulthood. Adulthood is marked by the demonstration of proper social behavior, a well-developed sense of responsibility, and the capacity to make socially and morally correct decisions. These characteristics are necessary to achieve the main goals of life, which are to create a family and a secure home and be able to support and nurture its members, both by taking care of necessities and by gaining a few comforts.

Perceptions about how to fulfill these life goals gradually change when immigrant families come to the United States and when U.S.-born Latinos are led to believe that they too can share in mainstream definitions of achievement and the "good life," which include higher social status and increasingly better income. In Chapter Five, we described how discouragement over lack of opportunity to attain this good life, according to mainstream American rules, can lead some Latino youth to reject secondary education and adopt an alternative and even deviant lifestyle. A study of academic invulnerability among tenth-grade Mexican American students supported the idea that certain resources and appraisals can buffer or protect at-risk students from situations that can lead to academic failure.[56] Chief among these resources is the educational support available from teachers and friends. Although other studies suggest that parental support is also vital, this study did not find an association between high grades and parents' educational support. Subjective appraisals seem most important as buffers against vulnerability for educational failure. Academically, invulnerable students felt prepared for college, liked school and its activities, had fewer conflicts with students in other groups, and had fewer family difficulties. In contrast, vulnerability was highly associated with language issues in relation to performance on tests of basic skills.

Normative Orientation: What Is the Right Way?

Practitioners working with youths need to be informed about rules and standards for behavior in local worlds. These are most often expressed in family life with the expectation that they will be adopted by the children. However, with the different levels of acculturation of parents and children, the expectation of many parents that family norms will be adopted goes unfulfilled more often than not.

Sexuality and Family

As already noted, in most if not all Latino cultures, girls are expected to be home-centered and to restrict their social relationships to relatives, close neighbors, and friends of the family. Reasons center on propriety and parental fears about sexual activity outside of marriage. (Ironically, in Puerto Rico a generation ago many marriages were arranged between cousins because of adolescent sexual activity.) Sexuality is a highly sensitive, taboo topic for pubescent girls and their parents, and if the taboos are not observed it leads to feelings of shame. In direct contrast there is a widely acknowledged (if not very openly discussed) sexual focus for boys, who translate sexual experience into self-esteem and a sense of manhood. In cohesive families, these experiences are usually acquired well beyond the home boundaries. Differential acculturation between daughters and parents creates considerable strain because of parental imposition of limits on teenage daughters who seek to avoid chaperonage and participate in European American ways of adolescent social life.

In the traditions of most of the countries of origin of U.S. Latino cultures, there has been no concept of dating before courtship and marriage. Heterosexual contact outside the family has traditionally been strictly monitored until a teenage couple makes a commitment to be *novios* (fiancés). Recent mainstream North American patterns, which condone social and sexual experience among unmarried youths or adults, are extremely uncomfortable for many Latino parents, especially fathers, who see their authority and protector role severely challenged when teenage daughters fail to respect them by becoming "loose" or "free" (prostitute-like) women. Moreover, parents rarely explain sex or contraception, inhibited by the view that an individual's sexuality is a very private matter not to be interfered in by parents or other family members. The dichotomy between private and public is also reflected in the custom that the general topic of sex may be burlesqued when the conversation is distanced from relatives and persons who are intimate (*de confianza*).

Family, Spirituality, and Ethos

Throughout this volume we have described many of the ways in which spirituality and religion are interwoven into the fabric of Latino life. In this chapter it remains to be said that the importance of spirituality to understanding the family is that it summarizes the ideals that family life should fulfill: wholeness, inner peace, interconnectedness, and reverence for life. For example, Latinos usually honor individual decisions by youth (even small children) about religious and spiritual preferences (although this is not as true for families who are members of Pentecostal churches) and do not insist on family-based mutuality in religious or spiritual behavior. This is part of a basic and fundamental respect for the privacy and individuality of a person's "soul" or inner life.[57]

When it comes to interventions, lack of family mutuality regarding religious activities can lessen the usefulness of church-based youth activities as substitutes for street gangs or other negative peer activities. However, a study of coping among ninth-grade students found that Mexican American youths reported using social activities and spiritual support significantly more often than did their European American peers.[58]

Family dynamics and interpersonal relations in the community should not be considered only from structural or behavioral perspectives but also in terms of affective style. Family psychologist Howard Liddle demonstrates the importance of understanding the "anatomy of emotions" in family therapy with adolescents.[59] Chapter Seven explores the impact of community relationships, which include affective reactions, on both the generation of and intervention in youths' problems. As we cautioned earlier, there are intracultural variations among Latino cultures, each has modal patterns of expressive style as well as cultural scripts on emotions.[60] Among Cubans there is a tendency toward high expressiveness characterized by flamboyance, exaggeration, and a love of a rich material life. Distress may not be disclosed until a relationship of trust (*confianza*) is established; but once this exists, distress is often communicated as a prolonged litany of despair, particularly by women. Psychologists Guillermo Bernal and Yvette Flores-Ortiz describe the sense of "specialness" that Cubans convey, not only verbally but also as themes in music, art, and literature.[61] Within virtually the same cultural heritage, Puerto Ricans have a similar, exuberant expressive style, but their approach to life is humbler. (This may be related to Puerto Rico's lesser historical and economic importance during the colonial period, and to its years of uninterrupted political domination by Spain and the United States.) In contrast, Mexicans are more reserved, perhaps because of their Indian heritage and their constant struggle to maintain a distinct cultural identity during centuries of close proximity to a powerful nation. Mexican Americans appear less reserved, but they too prefer to express their deeper feelings only to an inner circle of familiar confidants.

Initial assessment of either families or individuals is unlikely to tap these hidden feelings, which may only emerge when familiarity and trust develop. These perspectives on normative behavior, regarding appropriate affect, should be thought of only as generalized guidelines (that is, as things to observe or to inquire about) that can vary by age, gender, family culture, and individual temperament.

Conclusion

The goal of this chapter has been to offer an overview of those aspects of culture as context that are important to assessing, planning, and intervening into the social contexts that are the loci of the difficulties that Latino youths face. It is impossible to provide all of the aspects and implications of the cultural orientations of any one Latino culture in one short chapter, let alone cover the diversity of Latino groups. Where diversity seems especially important, as in traditions about an ancestral homeland, we have mentioned these differences in a more systematic way because they are important to the formulation of cultural identities and also affect ethnic identity as it develops in youths. Although far from comprehensive, if this chapter facilitates thinking about how to develop culturally responsive interventions and acts as a trigger for the further perusal of relevant literature (much of which we have cited), then our purpose will have been fulfilled.

Notes

1. C. Suarez Orozco and M. Suarez Orozco, "Migration: Generational Discontinuities and the Making of Latino Identities," in *Ethnic Identity: Creation, Conflict, and Accommodation*, 3rd ed., ed. L. Romanucci-Ross and G. De Vos (Walnut Creek, Calif.: Alta Mira Press, 1995), 341–347.

2. A. I. Hallowell, "The Self and Its Behavioral Environment," in *Culture and Experience,* ed. A. I. Hallowell (Philadelphia: University of Pennsylvania Press, 1955), 86.
3. S. L. Bem, "Gender Schema Theory: A Cognitive Account of Sex Typing," *Psychological Review, 88* (1981): 354–364.
4. J. M. Casas, B. R. Wagenheim, R. Banchero, and J. Mendoza-Romero, "Hispanic Masculinity: Myth or Psychological Schema Meriting Clinical Consideration," in *Hispanic Psychology: Critical Issues in Theory and Research,* ed. A. M. Padilla (Thousand Oaks, Calif.: Sage, 1995).
5. J. M. O'Neil, "Gender-Role Conflict and Strain in Men's Lives: Implications for Psychiatrists, Psychologists, and Other Human-Service Providers," in *Men in Transition: Theory and Therapy,* ed. K. Solomon and N. B. Levy (New York: Plenum, 1982), 5–44.
6. J. Finn, "The Relationship Between Sex Role Attitudes and Attitudes Supporting Marital Violence," *Sex Roles, 14* (1986): 235–244.
7. D. Castañeda, "Gender Issues Among Latinas," in *Lectures on the Psychology of Women,* ed. J. Chrisler, C. Golden, and P. Rozee (New York: McGraw-Hill, 1995), 167–182.
8. A. Hurtado, D. E. Hayes-Bautista, R. Burciaga Valdez, and A. Hernandez, *Redefining California: Latino Social Engagement in a Multicultural Society* (Los Angeles: UCLA Chicano Studies Center, 1992).
9. Castañeda, "Gender Issues Among Latinas."
10. Casas, Wagenheim, Banchero, and Mendoza-Romero, "Hispanic Masculinity."
11. H. Tajfel, *Social Identity and Intergroup Relations* (Cambridge, England: Cambridge University Press, 1982).
12. M. E. Bernal, D. S. Saenz, and G. P. Knight, "Ethnic Identity and Adaptation of Mexican American Youths in School Settings," in *Hispanic Psychology: Critical Issues in Theory and Research,* ed. A. M. Padilla (Thousand Oaks, Calif.: Sage, 1995), 71–88.
13. C. Markstrom-Adams and M. B. Spencer, "A Model for Identity Intervention with Minority Adolescents," in *Interventions for Adolescent Identity Development,* ed. S. L. Archer (Thousand Oaks, Calif.: Sage, 1990), 297.
14. M. E. Bernal and G. P. Knight, "Ethnic Identity of Latino Children," in *Psychological Interventions and Research with Latino Populations,* ed. J. G. Garcia and M. C. Zea (Needham Heights, Mass.: Allyn & Bacon, 1997), 15–38.
15. M. E. Bernal and others, "Development of Mexican American Identity," in *Ethnic Identity: Formation and Transmission Among Hispanics and Other Minorities,* ed. M. E. Bernal and G. P. Knight (Albany: State University of New York Press, 1993), 31–46.

16. J. S. Phinney, "A Three-Stage Model of Ethnic Identity Development in Adolescence," in *Ethnic Identity: Formation and Transmission Among Hispanics and Other Minorities,* ed. M. E. Bernal and G. P. Knight (Albany: State University of New York Press, 1993), 61–79.

17. Bernal and Knight, "Ethnic Identity of Latino Children."

18. Bernal and Knight, "Ethnic Identity of Latino Children."

19. M. E. Matute-Bianchi, "Ethnic Identities and Patterns of School Success and Failure Among Mexican-Descent and Japanese American Students in a California High School: An Ethnographic Analysis," *American Journal of Education* (Nov. 1986): 233–255.

20. E. Andujo, "Ethnic Identity of Transethnically Adopted Hispanic Adolescents." *Social Work* (Nov.-Dec. 1988): 531–535.

21. Bernal, Saenz, and Knight, "Ethnic Identity and Adaptation of Mexican American Youths."

22. L. H. Rogler, R. G. Malgady, and O. Rodriguez, *Hispanics and Mental Health: A Framework for Research* (Malabar, Fla.: Krieger, 1989).

23. L. M. Baca and J. D. Koss-Chioino, "Development of a Culturally Responsive Group Therapy Model," *Journal of Multicultural Counseling and Development, 25* (1997): 130–141; J. Szapocznik, M. A. Scopetta, and O. E. King, "Theory and Practice in Matching Treatment to the Special Characteristics and Problems of Cuban Immigrants," *Journal of Community Psychology, 6* (1978): 112–122.

24. Rogler, Malgady, and Rodriguez, *Hispanics and Mental Health.*

25. R. L. Harwood, J. G. Miller, and W. L. Irizarry, *Culture and Attachment: Perception of the Child in Context* (New York: Guilford Press, 1995).

26. D. Sewell, *Knowing People: A Mexican American Community's Concept of a Person* (New York: AMS Press, 1989).

27. Sewell, *Knowing People.*

28. A. C. Zentella, *Growing Up Bilingual* (Cambridge, Mass.: Blackwell, 1997).

29. Zentella, *Growing Up Bilingual.*

30. V. DiNicola, *A Stranger in the Family: Culture, Families and Therapy* (New York: Norton, 1997).

31. P. Bourgois, *In Search of Respect: Selling Crack in the Barrio* (New York: Cambridge University Press, 1995).

32. J. D. Vigil, *Barrio Gangs: Street Life and Identity in Southern California* (Austin: University of Texas Press, 1988).

33. Sewell, *Knowing People.*

34. B.S.G. Molina and L. Chassin, "The Parent-Adolescent Relationship at Puberty: Hispanic Ethnicity and Parent Alcoholism as Moderators," *Developmental Psychology, 32*(4) (1996): 675–686.

35. W. A. Vega, E. L. Khoury, R. S. Zimmerman, A. G. Gil, and G. J. Warheit, "Cultural Conflicts and Problem Behaviors of Latino Adolescents in

Home and School Environments," *Journal of Community Psychology, 23* (1995): 167–179.

36. P. Ruiz, "Cuban Americans: Migration, Acculturation, and Mental Health," in *Theoretical and Conceptual Issues in Hispanic Mental Health,* ed. R. G. Malgady and O. Rodriguez (Malabar, Fla.: Krieger, 1994), 70–89.

37. J. A. Garcia, "The Chicano Movement: Its Legacy for Politics and Policy," in *Chicanas/Chicanos at the Crossroads,* ed. D. R. Maciel and I. D. Ortiz (Tucson: University of Arizona Press, 1996), 85–86.

38. M. R. García-Acevedo, "Return to Atzlán: Mexico's Policies Toward Chicanas/os," in *Chicanas/Chicanos at the Crossroads,* ed. D. R. Maciel and I. D. Ortiz (Tucson: University of Arizona Press, 1996), 130–156.

39. García-Acevedo, "Return to Atzlán."

40. L. Comas-Díaz, M. B. Lykes, and R. D. Alarcón, "Ethnic Conflict and the Psychology of Liberation in Guatemala, Peru, and Puerto Rico," *American Psychologist, 53*(7) (1998): 778–792.

41. A. Lao, "Islands at the Crossroads: Puerto Ricanness Traveling Between the Translocal Nation and the Global City," in *Puerto Rican Jam: Rethinking Colonialism and Nationalism,* ed. F. Negron-Muntaner and R. Grosfoguel (Minneapolis: University of Minnesota Press, 1997), 169–188; A. Sánchez, "Puerto Rican Identity up in the AIR: AIR Migration, Its Cultural Representations, and Me," in *Puerto Rican Jam: Rethinking Colonialism and Nationalism,* ed. F. Negron-Muntaner and R. Grosfoguel (Minneapolis: University of Minnesota Press, 1997), 189–208.

42. Zentella, *Growing Up Bilingual.*

43. L. H. Rogler, D. E. Cortes, and R. G. Malgady, "Acculturation and Mental Health Status Among Hispanics: Convergence and New Directions for Research," *American Psychologist, 46*(6) (1991): 585–597.

44. Rogler, Cortes, and Malgady, "Acculturation and Mental Health Status," p. 591.

45. G. P. Knight and S. Kagan, "Acculturation of Prosocial and Competitive Behaviors Among Second- and Third-Generation Mexican American Children," *Journal of Cross-Cultural Psychology, 8* (1977): 273–284.

46. Vega, Khoury, Zimmerman, Gil, and Warheit, "Cultural Conflicts and Problem Behaviors."

47. M. Felix-Ortiz and M. D. Newcomb, "Cultural Identity and Drug Use Among Latino and Latina Adolescents," in *Drug Abuse Prevention with Multiethnic Youth,* ed. G. J. Botvin, S. Schinke, and M. A. Orlandi (Thousand Oaks, Calif.: Sage, 1995), 147–165.

48. T. La Fromboise, H.L.K. Coleman, and J. Gerton, "Psychological Impact of Biculturalism: Evidence and Theory," *Psychological Bulletin, 114*(3) (1993): 395–412.

49. J. Szapocznik, D. A. Santisteban, A. Perez-Vidal, W. M. Kurtines, and O. E. Hervis, "Bicultural Effectiveness Training," *Hispanic Journal of Behavioral Sciences, 8* (1986): 303–330.
50. La Fromboise, Coleman, and Gerton, "Psychological Impact of Biculturalism."
51. B. D. Ruben and D. J. Kealey, "Behavioral Assessment of Communication Competency and the Prediction of Cross-Cultural Adaption," *International Journal of Intercultural Relations, 3* (1979): 15–47.
52. K. Hakuta, "Distinguishing Among Proficiency, Choice, and Attitudes in Questions About Language for Bilinguals," in *Puerto Rican Women and Children: Issues in Health, Growth and Development,* ed. G. Lamberty and C. G. Garcia Coll (New York: Plenum, 1994), 191–209.
53. Vega, Khoury, Zimmerman, Gil, and Warheit, "Cultural Conflicts and Problem Behaviors," pp. 167–179.
54. Zentella, *Growing Up Bilingual.*
55. Zentella, *Growing Up Bilingual.*
56. S. Alatorre Alva, "Academic Invulnerability Among Mexican American Students: The Importance of Protective Resources and Appraisals," in *Hispanic Psychology: Critical Issues in Theory and Research,* ed. A. M. Padilla (Thousand Oaks, Calif.: Sage, 1995), 288–302.
57. Sewell, *Knowing People.*
58. E. P. Copeland and R. S. Hess, "Differences in Young Adolescents' Coping Strategies Based on Gender and Ethnicity," *Journal of Early Adolescence, 15*(2) (1995): 203–219.
59. H. A. Liddle, "The Anatomy of Emotions in Family Therapy with Adolescents," *Journal of Adolescent Research, 9*(1) (1994): 120–157.
60. A. Wierzbicka, "Cultural Scripts: A Semantic Approach to Cultural Analysis and Cross-Cultural Communication," *Pragmatics and Language Learning, 5* (monograph series, 1994): 1–24.
61. G. Bernal and Y. Flores-Ortiz, "Latino Families in Therapy: Engagement and Evaluation," *Journal of Marital and Family Therapy* (1982): 357–365.

Chapter Nine

Contextual Approaches: Practical Implications

At an early age, a ward of the system,
A product of his environment, a culprit, and a victim.
PLACIDO VASQUEZ JR.

We began this book with the case of Teresa, a client of a managed care system. The final outcome for Teresa was positive, thanks to her mother's being able to secure group therapy and individual counseling from a psychologist in private practice who was more responsive to the family's values and expectations than the HMO mental health provider had been. Subsequent to treatment with her daughter's new therapist, Teresa's mother no longer felt guilty about her "overprotectiveness"; instead, she felt ennobled by her deep concern for Teresa's well-being. As for Teresa, she again began to do well academically and for the first time in her life began to excel in track. Our contextual approach intends to remedy the kinds of difficulties that Teresa and her family initially experienced in seeking to obtain developmentally and culturally responsive mental health care.

In this concluding chapter, we will discuss four topics that we believe are central to the delivery of mental health services if a contextual perspective is adopted:

- Latinos' access to mental health services
- How managed care structures the way interventions are formulated and delivered, and the danger of the failure to take cultural diversity into account

- How the paradigms from which interventions are derived determine how cultural diversity is dealt with
- How the contextual approach we have described specifies a different, broader evaluation of interventions and changes the focus of determining the outcomes of treatment from models based primarily on quantitative methods to models including both qualitative and quantitative methods

Latinos' Access to Mental Health Services

The difficulties in providing developmentally and culturally responsive mental health care are compounded for the Latino working poor and immigrants who, unlike Teresa, do not have health insurance or the income to obtain private mental health care. Whereas nationwide about 15 percent of children under the age eighteen did not have health insurance in 1997, nearly 29 percent of Latino children were uninsured. This compared with 19 percent of African American children and 11 percent of non-Hispanic white children.[1]

On October 1, 1997, the State Children's Health Insurance Program (SCHIP), Title XXI of the Social Security Act, authorized $24 million over a five-year period to provide health insurance to low-income, uninsured children age eighteen and under who are not eligible for Medicaid.[2] This program promises to make mental health care services available to many previously uncovered Latino youth. Furthermore, SCHIP can be extended to school mental health services up to a certain percentage (although states may apply for a waiver to raise the limit).[3] Thus, SCHIP may provide a mechanism for previously uninsured Latino youth to access health care.

However, as mental health care moves into the schools to offer services where children spend most of their days, another problem becomes evident for Latino youth. Latinos, who now make up 13.5 percent of school-age youth in the United States, had an annual dropout rate in 1994 that was twice that of African Americans and three and a half times that of non-Latino whites.[4] In 1995, 30 percent of Latinos between ages sixteen and twenty-four either were not enrolled in high school or had dropped out.[5] Even when poverty, lack of English skills, and recent immigrant status are taken into account, the Latino dropout rate is still higher than for non-Latino counterparts with comparable backgrounds.[6] The dropout rate for

Latino youths born in the United States and speaking English at home is about 20 percent—again much higher than for these children's non-Latino and African American peers.[7] In future, when more mental health services will be offered in the schools rather than in off-site clinics, this high dropout rate will pose a problem not only because of reduced educational, career, and income opportunities for Latino youth but also because of reduced access to care for those youths who may have the greatest need. To reach these children, services will have to be community-oriented and neighborhood-based, such as those provided by the demonstration grants from the Center for Mental Health Services' Comprehensive Community Mental Health Services for Children Program, which we described in Chapter Seven.[8]

Managed Care and Contextually Oriented Interventions

Many mental health practitioners are unhappy with managed care. On the negative side, both the management of HMOs and the local and federal government call for "care for all" delivered in the same cookie-cutter fashion. Managed care delivery systems support this view by citing clinical research studies that show the efficacy of treatments described systematically in manuals, such as the use of cognitive-behavioral therapy for childhood phobias and adolescent depression. Organizing and delivering mental health care in a standard fashion is apparently considered the most cost-effective way, but it ignores the reality that clients are increasingly culturally diverse. Apart from the finding that there is a difference between treatment efficacy as measured in the clinical or laboratory situation and the effectiveness of the intervention in the real world (that is, the community settings where clients live), an equally serious problem must also be confronted.[9] The diverse cultural orientations of different groups, as well as the intragroup variations in culture, are rarely considered. As we have noted before, the gold standard of practice, treatment based on manuals, may be effective for clients for whom they have been designed: white European Americans primarily in the blue-collar and white-collar socioeconomic categories. However, the culturally different, particularly the unmeltable ethnics we described in Chapter One, are generally poorer, may speak other languages on a daily basis, and may have beliefs, values, and self-views and worldviews that generally are not considered under the standard treatments but may be crucial to the success of any treatment modality (through compliance, engagement, or retention in treatment). The idea that a standard array of empirically supported interventions developed for one segment of the U.S. population could be applicable to all clients is but another manifestation of the assimilation ideology that aims to eradicate cultural diversity from the United States. Unfortunately, in the case of standardized treatments, claims based on this kind of ideology are presented with presumed scientific validation.

On the positive side, another result of managed care's emphasis on cost effectiveness is prevention, which may lead to a public health approach to health care delivery. Prevention efforts bring the possibility that community mental health care might again become the focus of interventions and may open the way to modalities and programs framed by a contextual approach to intervention that seeks to incorporate both developmental and cultural responsiveness. A prevention orientation in mental health care is further spurred by *capitation,* the allotment of a fixed amount of money to a health care organization for a given client population for a given period of time no matter the amount, frequency, and type of services used by the client population. Once communities, rather than individual clients, are targets for the delivery of services, the need to understand population-based units and their subunits, such as the family, as well as interactions between persons and institutions in the community, will inevitably be given greater emphasis. Efforts to mount prevention programs in general can be associated with the realization that knowledge about the people in nonmainstream communities is necessary, because in order to prevent some undesirable state, whether physical or behavioral, those people must be "educated" or "persuaded" to accept the preventive interventions that health professionals expect will eliminate or ameliorate the problem.

A difficulty with this approach is the insidious tendency to view ethnic minority communities as rife with illness and problems despite statistics that demonstrate great variability in the prevalence of problems such as substance misuse, delinquency, and so on, both within and between Latino cultures in different regions of the United States. Immigrant communities are especially targeted for these types of judgments, even though some studies have shown that immigrant youth may be at least as healthy, behaviorally and emotionally, as youths born in the United States and perhaps even healthier.[10]

By denying health care to certain groups of immigrants or to undocumented workers, we are resorting to a political solution to our inability to develop effective, culturally responsive mental health care services. In part, this lack of culturally responsive services is the result of policies of cost containment in health care. These policies gain support more by popular sentiment than by knowledge of the actual costs of the delivery of services to these groups.[11] Unfortunately, the mental health of children of immigrants and undocumented workers has not been well investigated. And ironically, policies that exclude Latino immigrant and undocumented groups from receiving health care will undoubtedly hamper future research endeavors to understand better the mental health needs of these populations because they are not included in studies of populations receiving services.

Finally, a central issue in managed care is evaluating effectiveness of treatments. From the perspective of a contextual approach to interventions, the conundrum is obvious: If the treatments are not responsive to the characteristics, understandings, and expectations of those who receive them, then the evaluations of outcome are similarly unlikely to be valid. This view is certainly not unique; several movements within clinical child psychology have espoused it in different ways. A case in point is that of models of developmentally based, *integrated psychotherapy* with children, which advocate the tailoring of interventions to individual cases, as we have suggested earlier in this volume.[12] However, although they specifically incorporate developmental perspectives, integrative therapies are not contextual; they do not consider how culture patterns development within specific contexts. Even so, integrative therapies consider the importance of developmental differences among youthful clients, providing an important reason why a one-size-fits-all intervention is unrealistic.

Addressing Cultural Diversity

In the span of about twenty-five years, we have heard of the need to be "culturally sensitive," "culturally responsive," and most recently, "cultural competent." Numerous efforts are under way to develop and establish "cultural competencies" in the provision of mental health services by federal, state, and managed care organizations. Yet little attention has been given to the underlying assumptions that give rise to these terms. We have specifically avoided the use of the term *cultural competence* because it seems antithetical to a contextual perspective and has the potential to have political implications that we oppose.

Cultural Competence Versus Cultural Responsiveness

We mentioned earlier that cultural responsiveness, as we view it, does not include using interventions based on theories that by their very nature are not conducive to the consideration of culture. Rather, cultural responsiveness comes from developing interventions based on theories that incorporate culture in an integral way. The current exhortation in our professions to be culturally competent arises in part because the therapies we practice are not culturally relevant. Continuing efforts to adapt these therapies to include culture without embedding them in a paradigm that attends to cultural practices is unlikely to lead to effective treatment. Furthermore, the assumption that competence is the desired outcome in attending to culture in mental health practice seems to emphasize the technical rather than processual aspects of therapy. In a contextually oriented perspective that focuses on profiling the interactions between the individual, significant others, and multiple levels of context over the course of time, the therapist must attend primarily to process and secondarily to outcome.

Political Implications

The political consequences of practice models cannot be ignored. The central idea behind cultural competence is that practitioners must demonstrate the ability to apply a specific body of knowledge and skills to working with culturally diverse clients. Therefore, the practitioner in training can be evaluated based on level of cultural competence, according to the extent to which he or she can demonstrate use of these skills. If the standard of practice becomes cultural competence, then some mental health practitioners will be judged to be culturally competent and others will not. Many models for competency-based training—and even those leading to certification—adopted by professional organizations and state and federal agencies add cultural competence to their lists of competencies. Although this may provide some sense of justice for ethnic minority practitioners who believe that mental health practices have long ignored culture, the determination of cultural competence has in fact led to the institutionalization of "house ethnics."[13] House ethnics are ethnic minority practitioners in an organization or agency to whom ethnic minority clients are often referred. In professional organizations, ethnic minority practitioners frequently have been marginalized or compartmentalized in their own separate subgroups. For example, an organization may create a division, office, or committee for ethnic minority affairs to address cultural diversity in the profession. By doing so, these organizations inadvertently minimize the degree to which the general membership has to deal with issues of cultural diversity. As a result, professional organizations may be content to let a small minority of their membership become "culturally competent" while the majority disavows itself of the necessity to attend to culture in practice. As we discussed in Chapter One, culture is not just the property of those ethnic minority persons who do not assimilate to mainstream American society but rather is the universal human condition, and thus is at the very heart of therapy.

Significant Features of Contextually Oriented Interventions

A contextual approach, as we have described it, has several distinctive features. First, it views problems in terms of *poorness of fit* with respect to the youth in his or her environment and it formulates interventions based on how a youth's activity settings in different contextual levels can be altered or changed so as better to meet his or her developmental needs. Second, it emphasizes the role of the therapist as a consultant and collaborator with the parent and youth in mutually finding suitable solutions to problems rather than taking an expert's role in which the therapist prescribes a solution based on his or her preconceived notion of what will resolve the mental health problems of youth.

Third, our approach focuses on resources, strengths, and sources of support and protection in Latino communities in different environmental settings (such as the extended family or enhanced familism) as complementary to the framing of solutions to problems within those settings. Fourth, it stresses the need to recognize the impact of culture at each contextual level and its relation to the choice of interventions and how they are implemented in culturally responsive ways. It requires creativity and flexibility on the part of the practitioner to tailor the interventions to a particular youth-in-context. Finally, it demands that the practitioner appreciate the experience of the youth in varied activity settings across different contextual levels—for example, an appreciation of a boy's experience of power and effectiveness in his gang compared with the same boy's sense of hopelessness and impotence in his family, particularly when his drunken father abuses his mother.

Methods in Research and Practice

Psychology and psychiatry have strived to gain legitimacy in their companion fields. In so doing, many psychologists and some psychiatrists have emphasized using standardized, normative, behaviorally based assessments and applying quantitative methods to assess the efficacy of treatments. They advocate using empirically supported treatments (those with manuals are preferred) and place importance on fidelity in carrying out these treatments. Yet many practitioners in these two fields, as well as in social work and counseling, see mental health treatment as being more akin to the arts than to the sciences. Although some interesting innovations—such as narrative therapies that base their interventions on the constructed nature of knowledge—have much to offer in their applicability to culturally diverse populations, they have not yet been subjected to experimental scrutiny. These approaches may have more in common with literature and philosophy than such physical sciences as biology and chemistry.

The popularity of these newer social constructionist interventions suggests that there is a problem in using only empirical methods that derive knowledge about therapeutic outcomes by describing and comparing what *most* people do (that is, the numerical average) and then using this knowledge to understand what specific individuals do (that is, clients' behavior). One might argue that therapy could be guided or oriented by knowledge derived from statistical methods based on group means or averages; however, therapy is a change process that addresses a youth in relationship to others within diverse contexts. To understand this individual-in-context, we need clinical methods and assessments oriented to person-environment units.

It has been argued that qualitative and quantitative methods share common ground in four ways: they both detail evidence, they think about rival explanations, they seek results that are significant beyond the single study, and they demonstrate expertise in researching the subject at hand.[14] We suggest that both quantitative and qualitative research methods are required to examine the adequacy or effectiveness of contextual approaches such as the one we have described in this book. Although quantitative methods can be asserted to be comparative and generalizable, they suffer from a number of serious problems, especially from the perspective of the evaluation of a contextual model of intervention. First, they can only address certain varieties of subjectivity, and the decisions about which ones to address are based on theories that are imposed on the situation and settings to be evaluated. Experimental models attempt to control bias—such as in the selection of participants, for example—but generally cannot address certain types of bias that are common to treatment studies, such as an agency's priorities or an individual's preferences or responses to a particular type of intervention. As one evaluator notes: "Cronbach (1975) viewed the world of evaluation practice as one of complex contingencies and mediating factors operating in different contexts that are not adequately captured in main effects and producing interactions that do not generalize in patterned ways. But the study of these complexities requires that the evaluator be present and develop an understanding of the local conditions and of what makes the program work where it does work and impedes its effectiveness in other settings."[15]

Qualitative research ranges from exploratory to confirmatory (that is, it may seek to test or to explain further a conceptualization or construct).[16] Qualitative evaluation methods range in precision and comparative power from systematic descriptions of experiences, to mixed descriptions using observations, reports of experience, surveys and counts, and to case studies and experiential reports combined with surveys and questionnaires constructed on the basis of interviews with representative or key participants. Thus, the client-in-context can be adequately represented. In contrast, quantitative methods (in the case of treatment evaluation, most often quasi-experimental) when used alone minimize social and cultural context because they emphasize internal validity (reliability, or likelihood of obtaining the same results from different people) and generalizability (representativeness of most people's experiences).[17]

Contextual approaches emphasize the uniqueness of each person-in-context. Thus it is imperative that qualitative methods be used to describe fully what is happening and how the therapist intervenes across levels of context. However, we do not go so far as to say—as some social constructionists do—that each person's reality is unique and therefore cannot be compared with another's. Because we focus on culture as context we view a person's life much like a handwoven rug in which the strands represent the varied contexts. Just as no two rugs are the same, no two social constructions are the same. Yet Navajo rugs have commonalities even though each is somewhat different from the next. Indeed, the same can be said for Chinese or Persian rugs. In evaluating a contextual treatment, the uniqueness of each person's life and therapeutic experience (such as the youth's emotions when communicating with parents at specific times) can be examined by using qualitative methods, and those dimensions that can be seen to be common (such as patterned responses by the Mexican immigrant family to the practitioner or other official outsider, or frequency of drug use when in the company of certain peers) can be examined using quantitative methods.

Conclusion

We agree with Barbara Held when she says that therapists "need a clearer understanding of the structure of the theoretical systems they use to guide their practice," and we have attempted to provide that for our suggested model.[18] To determine if an approach such as the one we have described in this book is actually effective, it must be evaluated. Does the approach, when applied to diverse Latino youth from diverse cultures, yield positive results with some or all of these cultures or some or all of the youths in them? This book has intended to provide ideas for practitioners in sufficient detail to assist them in carrying out culturally and developmentally responsive, contextually oriented interventions. We are hopeful that treatment researchers will take up the challenge to evaluate this approach and explore the effectiveness of the components of this model of intervention for a diverse population of Latino—or other minority—youth.

Notes

1. U.S. Bureau of the Census, "Health Insurance Coverage: 1997. Table 5. Uninsured Children by Age, Race, and Hispanic Origin: 1997." [http:www.census.gov/pub/hhes/hlthin97/hi97t5.html], Sept. 28, 1998.

2. E. Garrison, J. McGrath, and P. Armbruster, "SCHIP Comes In for School Mental Health," *On the Move with School-Based Mental Health, 3*(1) (newsletter from the Center for School Mental Health Assistance, spring 1998): 1, 3.

3. Garrison, McGrath, and Armbruster, "SCHIP Comes In for School Mental Health."

4. L. Schnaiberg *[Education Week on the Web]*, "U.S. Report Tracks High Dropout Rate Among Hispanics." [http://www.edweek.org/ew/vol-16/], Feb. 11, 1998.

5. D. Viadero *[Education Week on the Web]*, "Hispanic Dropouts Face Higher Hurdles, Study Says." [http://www.edweek.org/ew/vol-16/], Aug. 6, 1997.

6. Schnaiberg, "U.S. Report Tracks High Dropout Rate."

7. Viadero, "Hispanic Dropouts Face Higher Hurdles."

8. "Factsheet: Comprehensive Community Mental Health Services for Children Program." [http://www.mentalhealth.org/child/ccmhse.htm], July 8, 1998.

9. J. R. Weisz and B. Weiss, "Assessing the Effects of Clinic-Based Psychotherapy with Children and Adolescents," *Journal of Consulting and Clinical Psychology, 57* (1989): 741–746; J. R. Weisz, B. Weiss, and G. R. Donenberg, "The Lab Versus the Clinic," *American Psychologist, 47*(12) (1992): 1578–1595; J. R. Weisz, G. R. Donenberg, and S. S. Han, "Bridging the Gap Between Laboratory and Clinic in Child and Adolescent Psychotherapy," *Journal of Consulting and Clinical Psychology, 63*(5) (1995): 688–701.

10. W. A. Vega, E. L. Khoury, R. S. Zimmerman, A. G. Gil, and G. J. Warheit, "Cultural Conflicts and Problem Behaviors of Latino Ado-

lescents in Home and School Environments," *Journal of Community Psychology, 23* (1994): 167–179.

11. L. R. Chavez, E. T. Flores, and M. Lopez-Garcia, "Undocumented Latin American Immigrants and U.S. Health Services: An Approach to the Political Economy of Utilization," *Medical Anthropology Quarterly, 6*(1) (1992): 2–26.

12. See S. W. Russ (guest ed.), "Special Section on Developmentally Based Integrated Psychotherapy with Children: Emerging Models," *Journal of Clinical Child Psychology, 27*(1) (1998).

13. The term *house ethnics* was coined by Jay Lappin in "On Becoming a Culturally Conscious Family Therapist," in *Cultural Perspectives in Family Therapy,* ed. C. J. Falicov (Gaithersburg, Md.: Aspen, 1983), 122–135.

14. R. K. Yin, "Evaluation: A Singular Craft," *New Directions for Program Evaluation, 61* (1994): 71–84.

15. See M. L. Smith, "Qualitative Plus/Versus Quantitative: The Last Word," *New Directions for Program Evaluation, 61* (1994): 39, in which Smith cites L. J. Cronbach, "Beyond the Two Disciplines of Scientific Psychology," *American Psychologist, 30*(2) (1975), 116–127.

16. M. B. Miles and A. M. Huberman, *Qualitative Data Analysis,* 2nd ed. (Thousand Oaks, Calif.: Sage, 1994), 17.

17. Miles and Huberman, *Qualitative Data Analysis,* p. 36.

18. B. Held, "The Antisystemic Impact of Postmodern Philosophy," *Clinical Psychology: Science and Practice, 12*(2) (1998): 264.

Index